AF625088

Heart Failure in Congenital Heart Disease

Robert E. Shaddy
(Editor)

Heart Failure in Congenital Heart Disease

From Fetus to Adult

Springer

Editor
Robert E. Shaddy
The Children's Hospital of Philadelphia
University of Pennsylvania School
of Medicine
Philadelphia, PA

ISBN 978-1-84996-479-1 ISBN 978-1-84996-480-7 (eBook)
DOI 10.1007/978-1-84996-480-7
Springer London Dordrecht Heidelberg New York

British Library Cataloguing in Publication Data
A catalogue record for this book is available from the British Library

Library of Congress Control Number: 2010937628

© Springer-Verlag London Limited 2011
Apart from any fair dealing for the purposes of research or private study, or criticism or review, as permitted under the Copyright, Designs and Patents Act 1988, this publication may only be reproduced, stored or transmitted, in any form or by any means, with the prior permission in writing of the publishers, or in the case of reprographic reproduction in accordance with the terms of licences issued by the Copyright Licensing Agency. Enquiries concerning reproduction outside those terms should be sent to the publishers.
The use of registered names, trademarks, etc., in this publication does not imply, even in the absence of a specific statement, that such names are exempt from the relevant laws and regulations and therefore free for general use.
Product liability: The publisher can give no guarantee for information about drug dosage and application thereof contained in this book. In every individual case the respective user must check its accuracy by consulting other pharmaceutical literature.

Cover design: eStudioCalamar, Figueres/Berlin

Printed on acid-free paper

Springer is part of Springer Science+Business Media (www.springer.com)

Preface

Survival outcomes for patients with congenital heart disease have greatly improved over the last two decades. Because of better and longer survival in these patients who often have abnormal ventricular morphology, the incidence of heart failure in this patient population has also increased. Although there is a significant evidence base for the treatment of heart failure in adults, the evidence base for treating children and adults with congenital heart disease is significantly less. The purpose of this book is to describe the current state-of-the-art for the diagnosis and treatment of heart failure in patients with congenital heart disease.

Contents

Contributors

Luis Antonio Altamira, MD
PediatricC ardiology,
The Hospital for Sick Children,
University of Toronto School of Medicine,
Toronto, Ontario, Canada

Charles E. Canter, MD
St.L ouisC hildren'sH ospital,
Washington University School of Medicine,
St.L ouis, MO,U SA

Scott R. Ceresnak, MD
LucilePa ckardC hildren'sH ospital,
Stanford University School of Medicine,
PaloA lto, CA,U SA

Konstantinos Dimopoulos, MD, MSc, PhD
RoyalB romptonH ospital,
SydneySt reet, London, UK

Troy E. Dominguez, MD
Great Ormond Street Hospital for Children,
London, UK

Anne Dubin, MD
LucilePa ckardC hildren'sH ospital,
Stanford University School of Medicine,
PaloA lto, CA,U SA

Michael A. Gatzoulis, MD,P hD
Professorof C ardiology,
National Heart and Lung Institute,
Imperial College,
London, UK

J. William Gaynor, MD
Departmentof S urgery,
The Children's Hospital of Philadelphia,
University of Pennsylvania
School of Medicine,
Philadelphia, PA,U SA

Georgios Giannakoulas, MD,P hD
RoyalB romptonH ospital,
SydneyS treet,
London, UK

Kimberly Y. Lin, MD
TheC hildren'sH ospitalof P hiladelphia,
University of Pennsylvania
School of Medicine,
Philadelphia, PA,U SA

Jack F. Price, MD
TexasC hildren'sH ospital,
Baylor College of Medicine,
Houston, TX,U SA

Chitra Ravishankar, MD
Pediatrics,T heC hildren's
Hospital of Philadelphia,
University of Pennsylvania
School of Medicine,
Philadelphia, PA,U SA

Andrew N. Redington, MB,B S,M RCP (UK), MD, FRCP (UK), FRCP (C)
PediatricC ardiology,
The Hospital for Sick Children,
University of Toronto School of Medicine,
Toronto, Ontario, Canada

Tami M. Rosenthal, MD
Divisionof C ardiothoracicS urgery,
The Children's Hospital of Philadelphia,
University of Pennsylvania
School of Medicine,
Philadelphia, PA,U SA

Jack Rychik, MD
TheC hildren'sH ospitalof P hiladelphia,
University of Pennsylvania
School of Medicine,
Philadelphia, PA,U SA

Robert E. Shaddy, MD
PediatricC ardiology,
The Children's Hospital of Philadelphia,
University of Pennsylvania
School of Medicine,
Philadelphia, PA,U SA

Deepika Thacker, MBBS
PediatricC ardiology,
The Children's Hospital of Philadelphia,
University of Pennsylvania
School of Medicine,
Philadelphia, PA,U SA

Heart Failure in the Fetus with Congenital Heart Disease

1

Deepika Thacker and Jack Rychik

1.1 Introduction

The cardiovascular system before birth is a unique, dynamic and complex organ system. In the fetus, physiological manifestations of the failing heart differ from that seen in the adult, child or infant for a number of reason. First, biological phenomena prior to birth can vary based on maturational changes that take place during different periods of gestation. Second, the diseases and ailments that afflict the fetal heart are of a different nature than that seen after birth and are unique to the developing human fetus. Finally, complex interactions take place between the developing fetus, its richly vascularized placenta and the supportive maternal circulation, creating a fascinating interplay of physiologies between the maternal mature and fetal immature systems.

In this chapter we review the tools used to assess the fetal cardiovascular system and discuss the pathophysiology and management strategies of a variety of disorders that lead to fetal heart failure.

1.2 Failure of the Fetal Heart: Physiological Considerations

The make-up of the fetal myocardium differs substantially from that of the mature myocardium. The fetal myocardium is comprised of approximately 60% non-contractile elements, as compared to 30% in the adult. The mechanism of myocardial calcium homeostasis at the level of the sarcoplasmic reticulum differs from that in the adult leading to slower reabsorption. Furthermore the fetal myocardium exists in a state of relative "constraint" with limited capacity for filling. The fetal lungs and pericardium exert a constraining force, in particular on the left ventricular myocardium, limiting ventricular cavity filling. With birth, the lungs

J.R ychik (✉)
The Fetal Heart Program, Cardiac Center at The Children's Hospital of Philadelphia,
34thStre eta ndC ivicC enterB oulevard, Philadelphia, PA 19104
e-mail:ryc hik@email.chop.edu

R.E. Shaddy (ed.), *Heart Failure in Congenital Heart Disease*,
DOI: 10.1007/978-1-84996-480-7_1, © Springer-Verlag London Limited 2011

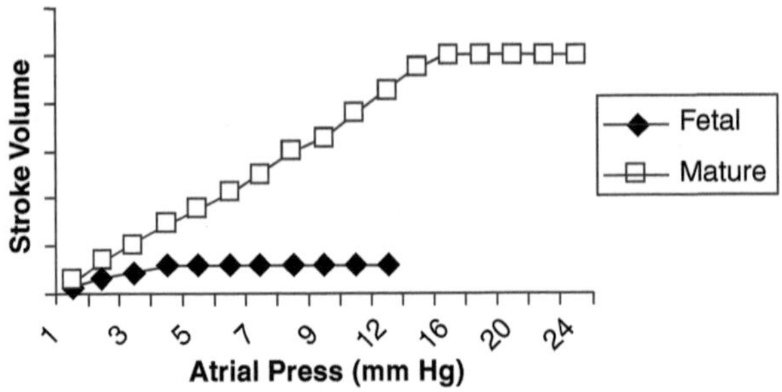

Fig. 1.1 Increase in ventricular stroke volume as atrial pressure rises with increasing preload. The adult heart can increase its stroke volume as preload increases up to atrial pressure of 16–18 mmHg. The fetal heart cannot increase its stroke volume beyond a peak occurring at approximately4–5m mHg

become aerated and expand, and are lifted off of the myocardium releasing the constraint and allowing for improved filling capacity. This takes place at the same time blood flow to the lungs and pulmonary venous return to the left atrium is substantially increased. Hence with the first breath taken at birth, two phenomena take place – an inherent capacity to accommodate a greater volume of blood by relief of ventricular constraint, and an increase in blood volume delivery secondary to increased pulmonary vascular perfusion.

All of these factors contribute to a relative stiffness of the fetal myocardium as compared to the mature heart leading to number of important considerations. First, under normal conditions, the ability to increase stroke volume is limited. In order to increase cardiac output, the fetus is very much dependent upon an increase in heart rate. Second, when conditions of disease are present the fetal myocardium has very little reserve. A comparison of the Frank-Starling curves of a fetal and adult myocardium demonstrates this point (Fig. 1.1). As ventricular filling increases, stroke volume increases linearly until a "break-point" is achieved at which point further filling does not lead to any further increase in stroke volume and the curve levels off. Due to the inherent "stiffness" of the fetal myocardium the break-point is achieved at a much lower filling pressure than in the adult. In essence, it takes very little to reach this break-point and achieve a state of inability to increase stroke volume in the fetus. This explains why many fetal cardiovascular disorders lead to the development of "hydrops," as increased ventricular filling pressure is very quickly transmitted back to the venous system.

1.3 Tools Used for Assessment of Heart Failure in the Fetus

Fetal ultrasound and echocardiography – including 2-dimensional and Doppler evaluation-have become integral to the assessment of cardiovascular compromise. Significant impairment of cardiac function in the fetus can lead to intrauterine growth retardation and abnormalities on general obstetrical assessments of fetal well being such as the "biophysical profile" (a composite assay of fetal activity and overall health). Elevation in central venous pressure secondary to cardiac dysfunction can lead to hydrops in the fetus, manifesting as fluid accumulation within the fetal extravascular compartments and body cavities, which can also be determined on obstetrical ultrasound assessment.

A detailed evaluation of cardiac anatomy is vital in the assessment of a fetus with suspected cardiovascular compromise. In addition, several measurements of cardiac function have been developed and refined since the initial descriptions of the echocardiographic assessment of the human fetus in the early 1980s.

1.3.1 Cardiothoracic Ratio

The fetal heart normally occupies one third of the fetal thorax. The cardiothoracic ratio can be calculated by measuring the transverse *diameter* of the heart at the level of the atrioventricular valves, or the *circumference* of the fetal heart and comparing it with the *diameter* or *circumference* respectively, of the fetal chest in the same image. This ratio is less than 0.5 in the normal fetus.[1,2] The cardiac to thoracic *area* ratio can also be calculated in a similar manner, and approximates 0.33 (range 0.25–0.35) (Fig. 1.2).[3–5] It is our practice to utilize the cardiothoracic *area* ratio as one can also easily make this assessment visually. In the normal fetus, one should be able to fit three hearts into the chest area. If one cannot visually place at least three hearts into the chest, then heart enlargement is present. The increase in heart size is an early marker in the fetus with compromised cardiac function. Enlargement and hypertrophy of individual chambers can be assessed by two-dimensional and M-mode techniques. The right atrium is the most common chamber to be enlarged in impending cardiac failure in the fetus.

1.3.2 Doppler Assessment of Atrioventricular (AV) Valves

Regurgitation of the atrioventricular valves is an indirect marker of cardiovascular dysfunction and can easily be identified by color Doppler evaluation of the fetal heart. Ventricular dilation with associated dilation of the valve annulus causes incomplete valve closure during systole leading to regurgitation. Any degree of mitral regurgitation at all and greater than trace tricuspid regurgitation is an abnormal finding in the fetus and indicates the need for further investigation.

Pulsed Doppler evaluation of mitral and tricuspid inflow patterns can provide clues to the diastolic status of the heart. After the first trimester, normal Doppler inflow patterns consist of two peaks, the earlier E wave representing passive early diastolic filling and the subsequent A wave representing filling with atrial contraction.[6] In the fetus, the E wave velocity is typically lower than A wave velocity reflecting reduced ventricular relaxation. Monophasic (single peak) filling of the ventricles is a sign of compromised diastolic function or severe external cardiac compression (Fig. 1.3). Changes in the E:A wave velocity ratios can be seen, but are variable depending upon the spectrum of etiologic factors present.[7–9]

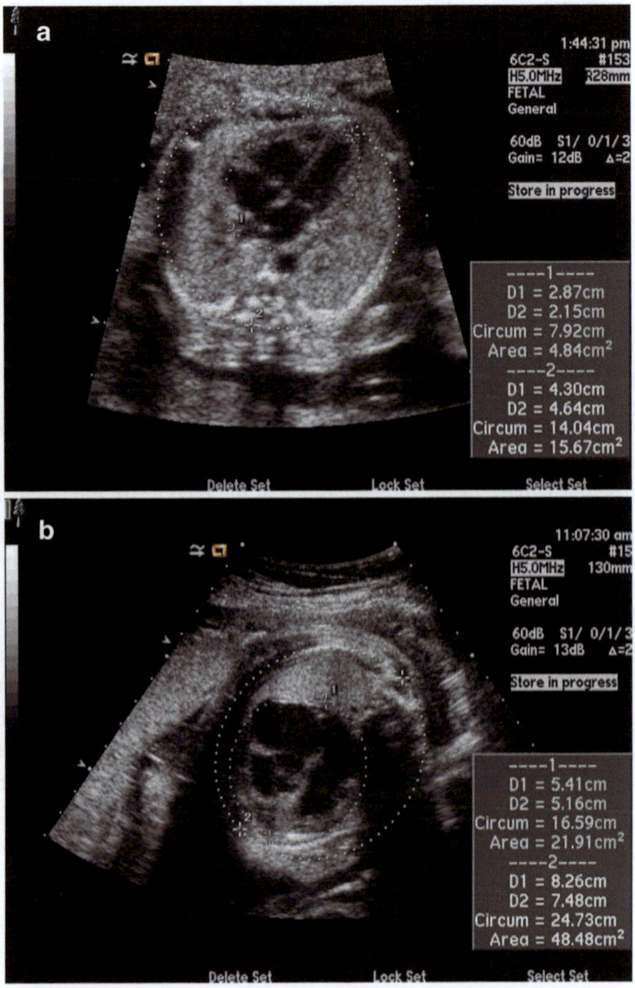

Fig.1. 2 Fetale chocardiogram showing the heart in a four chamber view with (**a**)norma l and (**b**)inc reased cardiothoracicr atio

1.3.3
Doppler Evaluation of the Ductus Venosus, Umbilical Vein and the Inferior Vena Cava

Fetal cardiac compromise results in elevated ventricular filling pressure and central venous pressure which in turn manifest as abnormal venous Doppler flow patterns in the ductus venosus, inferior vena cava (IVC) and the hepatic veins. While a reliable marker of cardiac dysfunction in the fetus with a structurally normal heart, changes in the venous Doppler flow pattern are also seen in right-sided obstructive lesions and complete heart block.

In the developing fetus, the ductus venosus shunts a significant majority of blood from the umbilical vein, directly to the IVC. Normal flow in the ductus venosus is low velocity and triphasic consisting of an S wave during ventricular systole; a D wave during

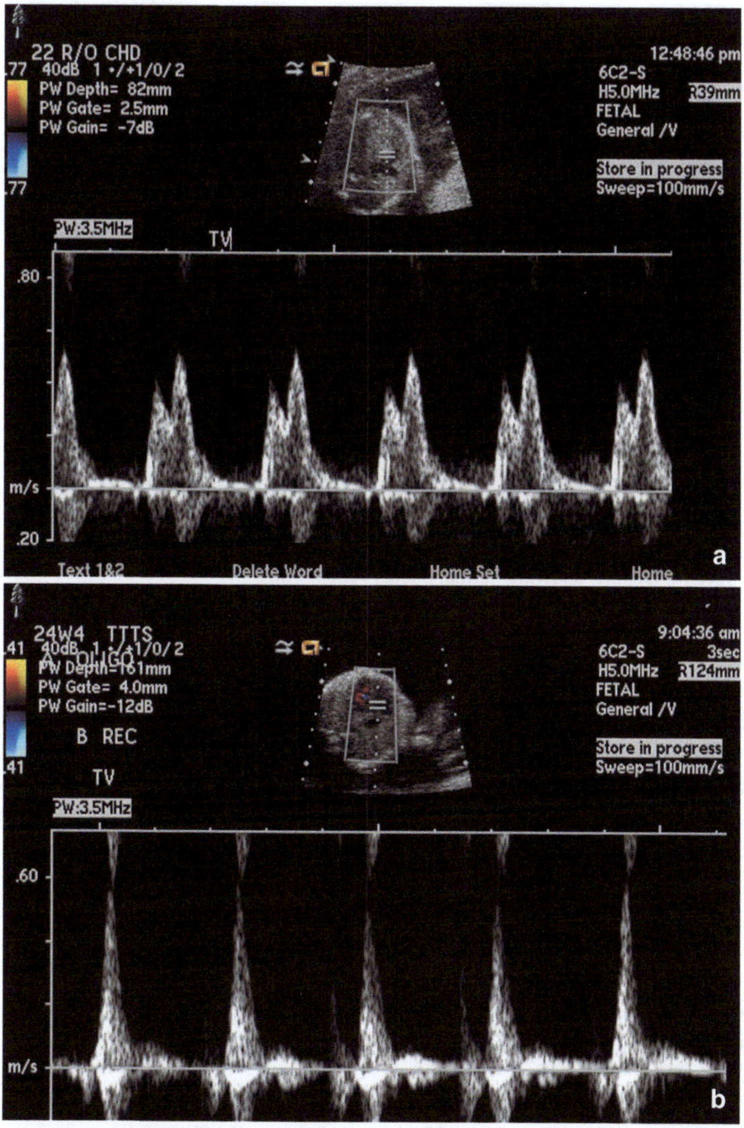

Fig. 1.3 Spectral Doppler evaluation of tricuspid inflow on fetal echocardiogram showing (**a**) normal and (**b**) single peak tricuspid inflowpa ttern

passive diastolic filling and an A wave during atrial systole.[10] Normally, blood flow in the ductus venosus is in the direction of the heart throughout the cardiac cycle (Fig. 1.4). Peak S, D and A velocities increase throughout gestation, although the S/D and S/A wave ratios remain essentially constant.[11] In the fetus with impaired cardiac function, increasing elevation of the central venous pressure manifests with progressively increasing

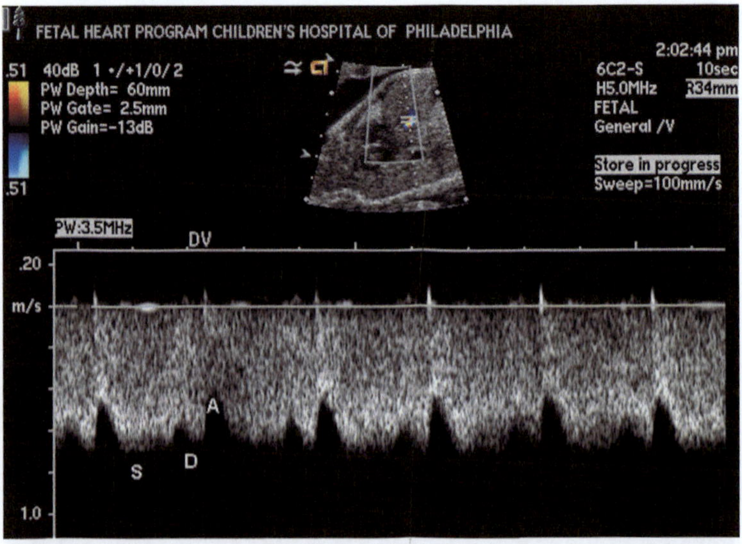

Fig. 1. 4 Spectral Doppler showing normal ductus venosus flow

reversal of flow during atrial systole (increasing A wave velocity) and decreasing D wave velocity (Fig. 1.5).

The flow in the IVC and the hepatic veins, similar to the ductus venosus, consists of a phasic low velocity pattern with S, D and A waves. In the normal fetus, there is a small reversal of flow in the IVC and hepatic veins with atrial contraction, producing an A wave which is in the opposite direction as the S and D waves. In the fetus with elevated central venous pressure, the magnitude of the flow reversal is increased.

Pulsed Doppler sampling of the umbilical vein in the central portion of the umbilical cord in the normal fetus consists of continuous low velocity forward flow with no pulsatility (Fig. 1.6). In later gestation, phasic variation with respiratory effort in the fetus is a normal finding. Fetal cardiovascular compromise with elevated central venous pressure results in notching of the continuous forward flow during atrial systole, thus producing a pulsatilepa ttern(Fig. 1.7).

1.3.4 Distribution of Blood Flow: Ratio of Resistances Between the Placental and Cerebrovascular Circulations

Regional blood flow in the fetus is influenced by multiple factors, including impedance of the distal vascular beds, structure of the heart, and cardiac output. In the fetus with placental insufficiency, some structural heart defects and in conditions resulting in low cardiac output, there is redistribution of fetal cardiac output due to a decrease in cerebral and an increase in placental vascular resistance. This is demonstrable as an increase in diastolic flow to the brain, a phenomenon termed as "brain sparing" – a physiological attempt to preserve blood flow to the vital organs such as the brain. This phenomenon can be

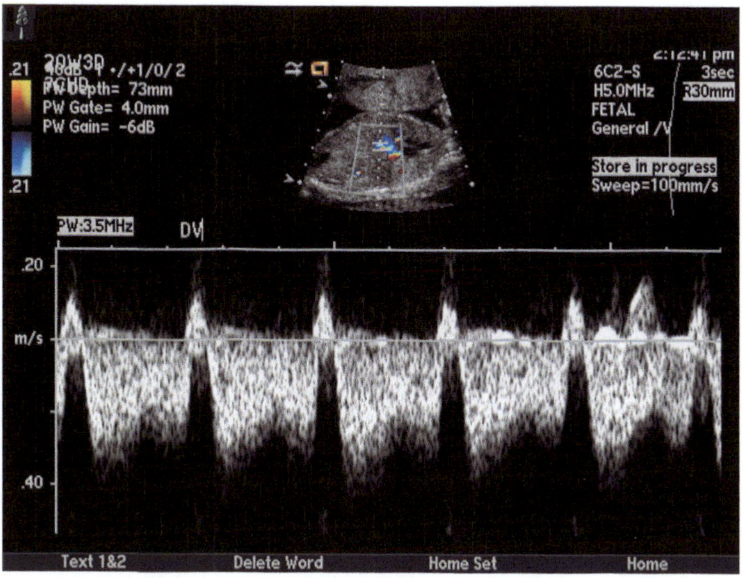

Fig. 1.5 Spectral Doppler showing abnormal flow reversal in the ductus venosus with atrial contraction

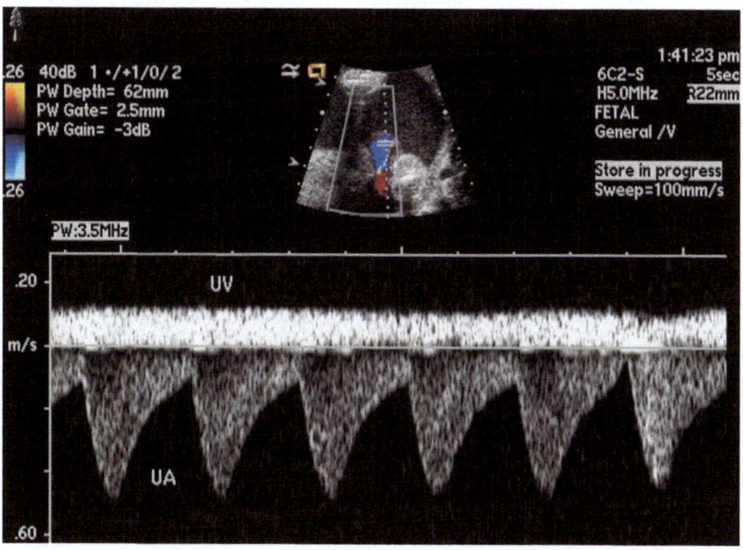

Fig. 1. 6 Spectral Doppler showing normal umbilical artery and umbilical vein flow

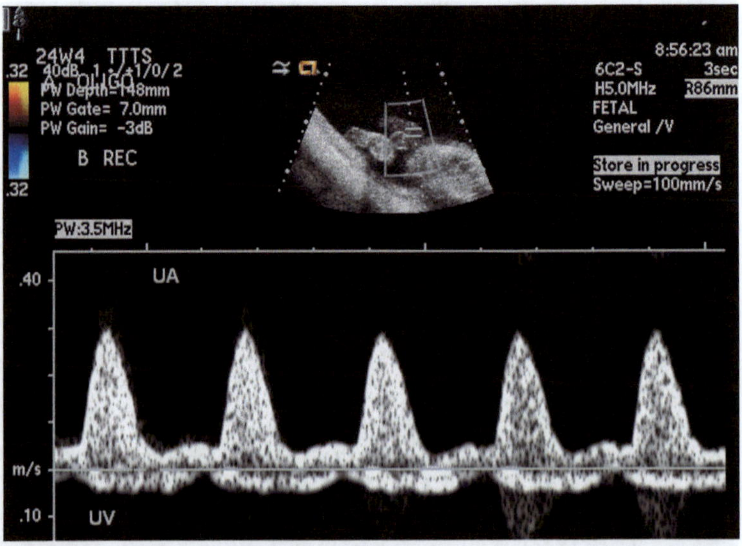

Fig. 1.7 Spectral Doppler showing decreased diastolic flow in the umbilical artery and abnormal flow in the umbilical vein with venous pulsations

quantified by evaluating flow in the umbilical artery (placental flow) and the middle cerebral artery (cerebral flow) and by looking at the ratio of vascular impedance between the two vascular systems. The ratio of cerebral/umbilical artery *resistance* and *pulsatility* has been shown to be a good measure of fetal blood flow distribution between the brain and the lower body and placenta. These changes may precede changes in the venous Doppler, and may thus be an important sign of early fetal cardiovascular compromise.

The *resistance* index (RI) and *pulsatility* index (PI) are both calculated using Doppler waveform tracings from the middle cerebral artery and the umbilical artery as follows:

RI = (peak systolic velocity – end diastolic velocity)/peak systolic velocity
PI = (peak systolic velocity – end diastolic velocity)/mean velocity

Several studies have shown that a cerebral/ umbilical pulsatility index ratio less than 1 is predictive for poor perinatal outcome.[12]

1.3.5 Estimation of Cardiac Output in the Fetus

Doppler echocardiography can be used to measure the cardiac output of the right and left sides of the heart and the combined cardiac output in the fetus.

Determination of the right and left ventricular output in the fetus requires: determination of fetal heart rate (FHR), velocity-time integral (VTI) of flow across the pulmonary and aortic valves, diameter of pulmonary and aortic valves (d) and estimation of the fetal weight. The individual ventricular output in mL/kg/min is then calculated using the formula:

$$\text{Output} = \{\text{FHR} \cdot \text{stroke volume}\,(\text{VTI}\cdot\pi\cdot d^2 / 4)\} / \text{estimated fetal weight}$$

The combined cardiac output (CCO) in the fetus is expressed as a sum of the left and right ventricular output with the right ventricle normally providing approximately 60% of the output. In the normal fetus CCO is approximately 425 mL/kg/min (range 425–550 mL/kg/min).[13,14]

Single assessment estimates of Doppler derived cardiac output can be fraught with error. Any small error in diameter measurement is compounded by the exponential nature of the formula used to calculate the valvular cross-sectional area and output. Consistent practice and meticulous operator care are necessary in order to master this skill. Nevertheless, we have found that serial measures of cardiac output in various disease states can be very helpful in monitoring the fetus in either gauging worsening state or in assessment of response to specific therapy. For example, conditions such as fetal anemia or arteriovenous malformations (AVM) can give rise to high output cardiac failure, and in these the CCO is markedly elevated except in very advanced stages of the disease. In conditions such as myocarditis, or when the heart is compressed such as in the presence of an intra-thoracic lung lesion, the CCO may be markedly decreased.

1.3.6 Assessment of Ventricular Performance

Estimation of myocardial function can be gauged in a very gross manner by looking at ventricular wall motion and quantification via measurement of either right of left ventricular shortening fraction. This can be a challenge as precise diameter measurements at a fixed specific anatomical site, a requirement for reproducibility, is much more difficult in the fetus than it is in the child heart. Some investigators have suggested the use of fractional area shortening as a better tool.

Several Doppler derived assays such as myocardial performance index (Tei Index) and Doppler tissue imaging have been reported. These tools have provided insight into the mechanisms of disease and may have clinical value in specific disorders when used in measuring changes in heart function in a serial manner.

1.4 Disorders of the Fetal Cardiovascular System and Heart Failure

1.4.1 Cardiomyopathy

Cardiomyopathy (CM) is defined as a disorder of the myocardium. Of cases diagnosed in utero, the vast majority are of the dilated type. Some metabolic disorders may present with hypertrophic CM in the fetus. The prognosis for fetal cardiomyopathy is understandably variable given the broad spectrum of underlying causes. In general, the presence of hydrops fetalis when cardiomyopathy is present is a poor prognostic sign usually leading to fetal demise.

1.4.2 Infection

Several infectious agents such as coxsackievirus, parvovirus, adenovirus, Epstein-Barr virus, toxoplasma, rubella, cytomegalovirus, and herpes simplex (TORCH agents) may cause direct myocardial damage with resultant dilated CM and heart failure in the fetus.[15] Untreated maternal syphilis and HIV infection may also result in fetal myocarditis.

Ultrasonographic findings such as intracranial and hepatic calcifications, hepatosplenomegaly and hyper-echoic bowel may point to an infectious etiology. The investigation of fetal myocardial dysfunction, with or without a maternal history consistent with infection, should include maternal hematologic indices and serological workup and, if indicated, amniocentesis and invasive fetal sampling to assess for anemia, thrombocytopenia, high specific IgM titers, viral cultures, and polymerase chain reaction for specific infectious agents.

Fetal therapy for myocarditis or CM associated with infection is presently only available in few conditions. Toxoplasmosis can be treated with pyrimethamine and sulfadiazine.[16] Penicillin therapy for syphilis may reverse the changes of congestive heart failure in the fetus. Corticosteroids and intravenous immunoglobulin (IVIG) have been tried in suspected fetal myocarditis though the benefits remains unclear.[17] Dilated cardiomyopathy in the fetus carries an extremely poor prognosis with a 55–83% likelihood of mortality or a postnatal course leading to neonatal transplant.[18–20]

1.4.3 Metabolic and Genetic Disorders

Maternal diabetes is the most common cause of hypertrophic cardiomyopathy and is manifested as ventricular septal hypertrophy in the fetus. Rarely, conditions such as glycogen storage disorders or Noonan syndrome in the fetus may present with hypertrophic cardiomyopathy.[21] Some metabolic disorders such as defects of carnitine metabolism may present as dilated cardiomyopathy.[22] Familial forms of cardiomyopathy, both dilated and hypertrophic, may have an in utero presentation.

1.4.4 Structural Heart Disease and Fetal Heart Failure

Structural heart disease in the fetus as a consequence of congenital malformation, for the most part does not result in heart failure. For example tetralogy of Fallot, transposition of the great arteries or even complex anomalies such as single ventricle and heterotaxy syndrome do not lead to heart failure in the fetus as myocardial function is typically normal. Although the intra-cardiac patterns of blood flow may be different than normal, and the potential for post-natal cyanosis and hemodynamic compromise following ductal closure are substantial in these anomalies, myocardial pump function in the fetus is preserved and ventricular filling pressures are normal, hence heart failure is not seen. However, a variety of forms of structural heart disease can lead to altered loading conditions, thereby resulting in heart failure. Structural anomalies with severe atrioventricular valve regurgitation, such as in common atrioventricular canal defect, Ebstein's anomaly of the tricuspid valve, or hypoplastic left heart syndrome with severe tricuspid regurgitation, may present substantially increased pre-load to the ventricular myocardium. Due to inherent limitations in capacity to accept any significant increase in pre-load in the fetal heart, heart failure and hydrops can readily develop in these.

Premature closure of the ductus arteriosus is a growing problem in the general population as an increasing variety of agents are being identified as potential stimulants for ductal constriction and possible closure. Non-steroidal anti-inflammatory agents (e.g. ibuprofen) and salicylic acid, as found in aspirin, are potent stimulants for ductal constriction in the fetus. In addition, a variety of herbal agents are suspected as possible stimulants to premature ductal closure. Premature closure or constriction of the ductus arteriosus can lead to increased right ventricle after-load, development of tricuspid valve regurgitation and may result in increased systemic venous pressure and in severe cases, hydrops. Treatment involves identification and elimination of the causative agent.

Tumors such as cardiac rhabdomyomas, or intracardiac or pericardial teratomas, may cause obstruction to ventricular filling by mass effect thereby altering pre-load, or cause outflow tract obstruction thereby altering after-load, which can lead to fetal heart failure.

1.4.5 High Output Heart Failure: Arteriovenous Malformation and Sacrococcygeal Teratoma

Vascular anomalies in which there is an abnormal connection between the arterial and venous system can result in excessive volume loading of the heart leading to heart failure. Initially there is a high cardiac output state as the heart compensates for the volume load with dilation and hypertrophy, meeting the increased demands of perfusion. However, with increasing arteriovenous shunting and progressive volume loading, myocardial stress increases and the myocardium itself begins to fail. As a consequence of ventricular dilation, atrioventricular valve annular dilation takes place leading to tricuspid or mitral valve regurgitation, further exacerbating the volume load.

Two anomalies that commonly lead to this pathophysiology are cerebral arteriovenous malformation (CAVM) and sacrococcygeal teratoma (SCT). In CAVM, the superior vena cava and carotid arteries are markedly dilated. Doppler interrogation of the aortic arch will reveal reversal of flow (retrograde flow) in the transverse and descending portion as a "steal" effect draws blood preferentially towards the lower resistance cerebral vascular circulation containing the CAVM. No fetal intervention is available for treatment of large CAVM, however digoxin can be used to assist in the management of significant fetal heart failure, if present.

SCT are large tumors that can grow to a size larger than the fetus itself. Oftentimes these tumors are highly vascularized and create a “perfusion sink” with increased venous return on volume load on the fetal heart. The inferior vena cava is typically quite dilated. An ominous finding is that of diminished or reversed flow in the umbilical artery, which suggests a lower vascular resistance for the SCT than for the placenta creating competition for blood flow from the descending aorta. In essence, diminished or reversed diastolic umbilical artery flow suggests that the SCT is stealing blood flow away from the placenta, a situation that will not permit for fetal survival. Currently, there are number of treatments available to treat fetal SCT including techniques for prenatal mechanical reduction of the vascular mass through injection of embolic material directly into the SCT. Open fetal surgery with SCT resection has also been attempted with some success. However, with either technique, the reduction of increased preload and sudden imposition of an increased afterload by elimination of the low resistance circuit, can cause serious cardiovascular instability.

Monitoring the fetus with CAVM or SCT via fetal echocardiography is critical for management. Serial evaluation for combined cardiac output is very helpful. The upper limits of normal for combined cardiac output in the fetus is approximately 500 cc/kg/min. We have seen fetuses with these anomalies achieve calculated outputs as high as 1,200–1,300 cc/kg/min. Combined cardiac outputs of approximately 750–800 cc/kg/min in the fetus are well tolerated, however outputs much beyond this value predict the development hydrops and fetal demise, in our experience. Hence a fetus with evidence for progressive increase in combined cardiac output, or the development of decreased, absent, or reversed diastolic umbilical artery flow demands fetal intervention or early delivery for postnatal surgical resection.

1.4.6
High Output Heart Failure: Fetal Anemia

Anemia in the fetus leads to a compensatory increase in cardiac output in order to maintain adequate tissue oxygenation. Fetal anemia can be induced immunologically as a result of a reaction between maternally produced antibodies and fetal red blood cell antigens, or non-immunologically as in fetal hemoglobinopathies.

The classic and most common type of immune mediated anemia is due to rhesus (Rh) alloimmunization. Kell antigen sensitization is the next most common type. Hydrops due to ABO alloimmunization is extremely rare but has been reported in the literature. One of the common causes of non-immune anemia is homozygous alpha-thalassemia (Hb Bart). It is an autosomal recessive condition with a 25% recurrence risk and is seen more commonly in the Southeast Asian population. When present it is uniformly fatal as fetal oxygen carrying capacity is progressively eliminated resulting in massive fetal hydrops. Other causes of non-immune anemia in the fetus include abnormalities of red cell production such as pure red cell aplasia, parvovirus infection, congenital leukemia and aplastic anemia; or red cell enzyme deficiencies such as glucose-6-phosphate dehydrogenase (G6PD) and pyruvate kinase (PK) deficiency.

Progressive anemia from any etiology leads to decreased blood viscosity. This results in increased peak systolic flow velocity in various parts of the fetal arterial and venous circulation.[23,24] One of the earliest signs of fetal anemia and impending heart failure is an increase in peak systolic velocity in the middle cerebral artery, which will occur *before* the increase in diastolic flow that reflects brain sparing when overt heart failure is present. Hydrops is a sign of very severe anemia and overt cardiac failure in these fetuses. Enlargement of the heart, liver and spleen, though not specific for anemia, may also provide clues to an earlier diagnosis.

Therapy for anemia in the fetus is possible and is directed towards the specific etiology. Immuno-modulation in the mother with plasmapheresis and intravenous immunoglobulin may be beneficial in management of anemia from Rh alloimmunization.[25] Hemoglobin Bart's, the most severe form of alpha thalassemia, is uniformly fatal in the fetal or immediate postnatal period. In cases such as severe anemia from Rh alloimmunization or parvovirus infection, intrauterine blood transfusion is possible and can be administered through the umbilical cord or the hepatic vein.

1.4.7 Fetal Heart Failure in Multiple Gestation Pregnancy

As a consequence of an explosion in knowledge concerning assisted reproductive technologies, the incidence of twin gestation is increasing. Two disorders, which may affect the cardiovascular system leading to heart failure, are seen in monochorionic (shared single placenta) twins. The twin-twin transfusion syndrome (TTTS) occurs when there are vascular connections within the placenta, which cause a net volume of flow from one twin (donor) to the other (recipient), leading to a cascade of physiological effects. As the donor twin experiences hypovolemia, there is upregulation of its renin-angiotensin system with release of vasoconstrictive mediators aimed at maintaining perfusion. The recipient twin receives the volume load from the donor, however it also receives the vasoconstrictive mediators released by the donor. This combination of volume load and abnormal hormonal factors delivered to the recipient twin lead to a progressive cardiomyopathy, which can be observed via fetal echocardiography. Findings such as ventricular dilation, hypertrophy, systolic dysfunction, and AV valve regurgitation are common ultimately leading to heart failure, hydrops and fetal demise in some. Doppler echocardiography can reveal early subtle changes in this process. Specifically we have identified the presence of a single peak inflow pattern (whereas double peak is normal) in the right ventricle of recipient twins, with further changes in the ductus venosus and umbilical vein in those with progressive disease. No such cardiovascular changes take place in the donor, however observation reveals small ventricular cavity volumes in some and a decrease in the umbilical artery diastolic flow reflecting elevated placental vascular resistance. A 20 point scoring system highlighting each of the cardiovascular elements that manifest in TTTS has been developed by our group, and is used to help gauge the need for intervention and response to therapy.[26] The most effective current therapy is laparoscopic laser photocoagulation of the placental vascular anastomoses, which when successful, can reverse many of the cardiovascular findings in the recipient twin.

A second disorder seen in twin gestation is the rare finding of the "twin reverse arterial perfusion (TRAP)" sequence. This is a phenomenon that occurs in the presence of a monochorionic twin pregnancy, but where one twin is acardiac, or absent a well formed functioning heart. The acardiac twin acts as a biological mass that is supported by its normal twin partner, adding a volume load to the normal twin heart. The effect on the normal twin heart is similar to that seen in SCT or AVM. The term "TRAP" refers to the fact that umbilical artery perfusion of the "acardiac" twin occurs in a reverse manner – from placenta to fetus, as opposed to from fetus to placenta – as the normal twin perfuses the acardiac through placental vascular connections. Combined cardiac output in the normal twin of TRAP sequence can be increased leading to heart failure. When present, interruption of cord flow to the acardiac twin through cord coagulation or other techniques will eliminate flow, reducing volume load and preventing or reversing heart failure in the normal twin.

1.4.8 Fetal Heart and Maternal Diabetes

Maternal gestational diabetes is on the rise as a consequence of the increasing prevalence of overweight and obese mothers in the United States today. Although conventionally thought to be an isolated disorder of glucose metabolism, diabetes is in reality a pervasive disorder of metabolic derangement affecting glucose, fatty acid, and protein processing with far reaching effects on the developing fetus. Despite improvements in obstetric and perinatal care, pregnancies associated with maternal diabetes carry a significantly higher risk of fetal and neonatal complications. With maternal diabetes, the risk of major congenital malformations are two to ten times higher than normal pregnancies.[27–29] Studies report a 3–5% risk of structural heart disease in the fetuses of diabetic mothers, the predominant lesions reported being ventricular septal defects and conotruncal anomalies including transposition of the great arteries, tetralogy of Fallot, truncus arteriosus and double-outlet right ventricle.[27,30]

Aside from significant structural anomalies, fetuses of diabetic mothers carry an almost 30% risk of hypertrophic cardiomyopathy with disproportionate septal hypertrophy.[31] Morphologic changes of myocardial hypertrophy can be detected by fetal echocardiography in mid-gestation and may progressively worsen to term. While these changes tend to be more severe with poor maternal diabetic control, studies have shown structural myocardial changes and increased inter-ventricular septal thickness even in fetuses with well controlled maternal diabetes.[32] Most cases of myocardial hypertrophy secondary to maternal diabetes, are non obstructive and tend to resolve in infancy following separation from the maternal metabolic stimulus. However, there are reports of sudden death in utero or in the perinatal period attributed to this condition.

Systolic and diastolic cardiac function is usually preserved in fetuses with mild septal hypertrophy and well-controlled maternal diabetes. However, severe fetal and neonatal hypertrophic cardiomyopathy, in the setting of maternal diabetes may be associated with significantly increased ventricular stiffness and diastolic dysfunction, or outflow tract obstruction. Frank congestive heart failure and fetal hydrops is a rare finding.

1.4.9 Fetal Arrhythmia and Heart Failure

Fetal arrhythmias, either fast or slow, can cause heart failure during gestation. Fetal tachycardia occurs in approximately 0.5% of all pregnancies.[33] Normal fetal heart rate is between

110 and 160 bpm. Temporary accelerations in heart rate are a normal finding in the fetus. These are characterized by gradual onset and cessation and are usually under 200 bpm. Rates greater than 210 bpm are always abnormal.

The fetal tachyarrhythmias can be sub-classified according to their origin and mechanism, similar to the classification of postnatal tachyarrhythmias. Of the cases of supraventricular tachycardia (SVT), the most common form is atrioventricular reentrant tachycardia (AVRT) which accounts for 60–80% of cases. Atrial flutter accounts for approximately 20% of cases. Ectopic atrial tachycardia and multifocal tachycardia are rare and account for less than 1% of fetal SVT. Junctional ectopic tachycardia (JET) and ventricular tachycardia, while rare, are associated with poor outcomes and usually require therapy regardless of the ventricular rate.

Detailed analysis of the type of tachyarrhythmia in utero is possible using M-mode and Doppler echocardiography. In particular, a simultaneous record of Doppler waveform at the superior venous cava and the ascending aorta is an important and useful method of assessing the interval between atrial and ventricular contractions. With the introduction of myocardial deformation imaging using tissue velocity or strain rate analysis, these tachyarrhythmias can now be diagnosed more accurately. It is technically possible to record the electrical activity of the fetal heart across the mother's abdomen using sophisticated signal processing techniques. Fetal electrocardiography (FECG) is based on signal averaging of electrical signals but is not useful in arrhythmias with an irregular heart rate. Fetal magnetocardiography (FMCG) provides better signal transmission but is limited by the need for expensive equipment and a magnetically shielded room.

Sustained fetal tachyarrhythmias lead to foreshortening of the diastolic filling time, thus increasing the end diastolic pressure in the fetal atria. This manifests as hydrops in the fetus even before signs of ventricular systolic dysfunction become evident. Almost 40% of fetuses with SVT and atrial flutter develop hydrops in utero.

Due to relatively low toxicity, maternal digoxin is often used as first line therapy in the management of fetal SVT and atrial flutter. Oral or intravenous maternal loading is used when hydrops is absent as trans-placental transfer is relatively high. Direct intramuscular fetal injection may be used if there is hydrops, in order to avoid problems related to poor placental transfer. Conversion rates in response to digoxin are in the range of 50–60% for fetal SVT and approximately 45–50% for atrial flutter, though these are greatly reduced in the presence of fetal hydrops.[34,35] Maternal therapy with sotalol, which is a class III antiarrhythmic agent, is increasingly being used either alone or in combination with digoxin.[36] Of note, there have been reports of sudden fetal death related to sotalol presumable secondary to its proarrhythmic effect and fetal torsades de pointes. Amiodarone, another class III antiarrhythmic agent, may be used in resistant cases. However significant side effects, especially fetal and maternal hypothyroidism can be a limiting factor in its use.[37] Flecainide is a class IC antiarrhythmic agent with overall good transplacental transfer and is especially useful in the hydropic fetus with SVT, either alone or in combination with digoxin.[38,39] Direct fetal treatment with adenosine or other agents with injection into the umbilical vein or the right ventricle may be attempted in resistant cases of fetal SVT.[39]

Bradycardia, in the form of heart block can also cause serious heart failure in the fetus. Isolated complete heart block in the fetus is most commonly seen in the setting of maternal autoantibodies to SSB/La or SSA/Ro ribonucleoproteins. Almost 2% of pregnant women are believed to carry these antibodies, many of them without any manifestations of a connective tissue disorder. Of these, 1–2% of their fetuses will develop complete heart block typically between 18 and 24 weeks of gestation.[40] When heart block occurs, the fetal ventricular escape rate is usually around 55–60 bpm, however it can be as low as in the 30 s, this while the atrial rate remains normal at 110–160 bpm. An increased atrial rate in the presence of complete heart block may reflect a compensatory atrial tachycardia as the fetus attempts to maintain cardiac output.

The diagnosis of fetal heart block is established by demonstration of atrioventricular dissociation on fetal echocardiography by M-mode, pulse wave Doppler, or tissue Doppler imaging. Fetal electrocardiography and FMCG are now used to establish the diagnosis in some centers.[41,42] Myocarditis, endocardial fibroelastosis and dilated cardiomyopathy are also commonly seen in association with maternal autoimmune heart block, or in fact can occur independent of the heart block. Selective maternal antibody destruction of the conduction tissue with selectivity for the AV node is the believed mechanism for development of heart block. However, at times these same antibodies attack the myocardium directly causing inflammation and myocarditis, in the absence of heart block.

A low heart rate in the fetus with complete heart block leads to prolonged diastolic filling of the ventricle. The limited compliance of the fetal myocardium results in increased diastolic pressure with even a small increase in diastolic filling volume. This phenomenon, along with elevated right atrial pressure due to atrioventricular asynchrony with atrial contraction against a closed atrioventricular valve, predisposes to the development of fetal hydrops. Furthermore, the fetus is highly dependent on heart rate to maintain adequate cardiac output. With complete heart block, there is a very slight but limited compensatory increase in the stroke volume by ventricular dilation and hypertrophy. However, when heart rates are lower than 55 bpm there is a high risk of low cardiac output with subsequent poor tissue perfusion and fetal or perinatal demise.

Without fetal therapy, the mortality for maternal autoimmune complete heart block depends upon the ventricular rate achieved, but ranges from 18% to 43%.[43,44] Fluorinated steroids, most commonly dexamethasone are administered to the mother starting from the time of diagnosis of any degree of atrioventricular conduction delay in the antibody-exposed fetus. There is mounting evidence that treatment with fluorinated steroids may perhaps resolve incomplete heart block, although this remains controversial.[45] Unfortunately, the progression to complete heart block is typically quite rapid and most fetuses when diagnosed have established complete heart block. While damage to the atrioventricular conduction tissue is irreversible at this stage, dexamethasone has shown to help in improvement in myocardial function and hydrops, presumably related to its anti-inflammatory properties and potential protection of the myocardium from further inflammatory damage.[45] High dose beta-stimulant medications such as oral albuterol are recommended for fetal heart rates under 55 bpm. Maternal plasma exchange, maternal immunoglobulin therapy and azathioprine have been tried in some reports, but carry a high risk to both the mother and the fetus. Most babies born with congenital complete heart block require placement of an epicardial pacemaker in the first few months of life.

Heart block may also be associated with structural heart disease, most commonly corrected transposition of the great arteries (L-transposition, {S,L,L}) and polysplenia type of heterotaxy syndrome. Occasionally it can also be seen in simple atrioventricular canal defect.

1.4.10 Other Causes of Fetal Heart Failure

Fetal asphyxia can result in direct myocardial damage and cardiac decompensation. Endocardial fibroelastosis is a rare condition resulting from pathologic deposition of elastic and fibrous tissue within the endocardium and can occur as a non-specific response to a variety of pathological stimuli. It may occur in association with left sided obstructive lesions, viruses (mumps), genetic causes or fetal asphyxia and lead to a presentation of severe diastolic dysfunction and restrictive cardiomyopathy. Most fetuses die in utero or in the early neonatal period in those in which it is acquired and not part of structural congenital heart disease.

1.4.11 Maternal Complications of Heart Failure in the Fetus

In additional to a poor prognosis for the fetus, there are maternal complications associated with severe compromise of fetal cardiac function and hydrops fetalis. These complications include maternal anemia, pregnancy-induced hypertension, and antepartum hemorrhage. Complications such as abnormal presentation, prematurity, non-reassuring fetal heart rate pattern, and difficult vaginal delivery can lead to a higher cesarean delivery rate in these patients. Retained placenta and postpartum hemorrhage also are more frequent in these patients. Patients with an early onset of hypertension or polyhydramnios should heighten the suspicion, and a detailed assessment of fetal cardiovascular status should be performed in these cases.

1.5 Conclusion

Heart failure in the fetus can occur due to a variety of disorders that are unique and differ from the spectrum of disorders causing heart failure seen in the child or young adult. Not only are the causes of heart failure different, but the response of the immature fetal myocardium is different as well. Echocardiography provides a set of tools that helps decipher the pathophysiology of these complex disorders, however much more knowledge is necessary to fully understand these complex mechanisms. Once our understanding of the pathophysiology improves, we can then begin to implement management strategies and therapies currently lacking, that will optimize outcome for the fetus and its postnatal life ahead.

References

1. Tongsong T, Wanapirak C, Sirichotiyakul S, Piyamongkol W, Chanprapaph P. Fetal sonographic cardiothoracic ratio at midpregnancy as a predictor of Hb Bart disease. *J Ultrasound Med.*1999;18:807–81 1.
2. Paladini D, Chita SK, Allan LD. Prenatal measurement of cardiothoracic ratio in evaluation of heart disease. *Arch Dis Child.*1990; 65:20–23.
3. Shaw SL. Fetal Cardiomyopathies. In: Drose, ed. *Fetal Echocardiography*. Philadelphia, PA: Saunders;1998:263–277.
4. Chaoui R, Bollmann R, Goldner B, Heling KS, Tennstedt C. Fetal cardiomegaly: echocardiographic findings and outcome in 19 cases. *Fetal Diagn Ther.*1994; 9:92–104.
5. Respondek M, Respondek A, Huhta JC, Wilczynski J. 2D echocardiographic assessment of the fetal heart size in the 2nd and 3rd trimester of uncomplicated pregnancy. *Eur J Obstet Gynecol Reprod Biol.*1992; 44:185–188.
6. Makikallio K, Jouppila P, Rasanen J. Human fetal cardiac function during the first trimester of pregnancy. *Heart.*2005; 91:334–338.
7. Barrea C, Alkazaleh F, Ryan G, McCrindle BW, Roberts A, Bigras JL et al. Prenatal cardiovascular manifestations in the twin-to-twin transfusion syndrome recipients and the impact of therapeutic amnioreduction. *Am J Obstet Gynecol.*2005; 192:892–902.
8. Tsyvian P, Malkin K, Artemieva O, Wladimiroff JW. Assessment of left ventricular filling in normally grown fetuses, growth-restricted fetuses and fetuses of diabetic mothers. *Ultrasound Obstet Gynecol.*1998; 12:33–38.
9. Wong SF, Chan FY, Cincotta RB, McIntyre HD, Oats JJ. Cardiac function in fetuses of poorly-controlled pre-gestational diabetic pregnancies-a pilot study. *Gynecol Obstet Invest.* 2003;56:113–116.
10. Huhta JC. Guidelines for the evaluation of heart failure in the fetus with or without hydrops. *Pediatr Cardiol.* 2004;25:274–286.
11. Axt-Fliedner R, Wiegank U, Fetsch C, Friedrich M, Krapp M, Georg T et al. Reference values of fetal ductus venosus, inferior vena cava and hepatic vein blood flow velocities and waveform indices during the second and third trimester of pregnancy. *Arch Gynecol Obstet.* 2004;270:46–55.
12. Arbeille P, Body G, Saliba E, Tranquart F, Berson M, Roncin A et al. Fetal cerebral circulation assessment by Doppler ultrasound in normal and pathological pregnancies. *Eur J Obstet Gynecol Reprod Biol.*1988; 29:261–273.
13. Mielke G, Benda N. Cardiac output and central distribution of blood flow in the human fetus. *Circulation.*2001 ;103:1662–1668.
14. De Smedt MC, Visser GH, Meijboom EJ. Fetal cardiac output estimated by Doppler echocardiography during mid- and late gestation. *Am J Cardiol.*1987; 60:338–342.
15. Wagner HR. Cardiac disease in congenital infections. *Clin Perinatol.*1981; 8:481–497.
16. Remington J, McLeod R, Thuilliez P, Desmonts G. Toxoplasmosis. In: Remington J, Klein J, Wilson C, Baker C, eds. *Infectious Diseases of the Fetus and Newborn Infant.* 6th ed. Philadelphia, PA: Elsevier Saunders; 2006:947–1091.
17. Pedra SR, Smallhorn JF, Ryan G, Chitayat D, Taylor GP, Khan R et al. Fetal cardiomyopathies: pathogenic mechanisms, hemodynamic findings, and clinical outcome. *Circulation.* 2002;106:585–591.
18. Pedra SR, Hornberger LK, Leal SM, Taylor GP, Smallhorn JF. Cardiac function assessment in patients with family history of nonhypertrophic cardiomyopathy: a prenatal and postnatal study. *Pediatr Cardiol.*2005; 26:543–552.
19. Schmidt KG, Birk E, Silverman NH, Scagnelli SA. Echocardiographic evaluation of dilated cardiomyopathy in the human fetus. *Am J Cardiol.*198 9;63:599–605.

20. Yinon Y, Yagel S, Hegesh J, Weisz B, Mazaki-Tovi S, Lipitz S et al. Fetal cardiomyopathy-in utero evaluation and clinical significance. *Prenat Diagn.*2007; 27:23–28.
21. Burwinkel B, Scott JW, Buhrer C, van Landeghem FK, Cox GF, Wilson CJ et al. Fatal congenital heart glycogenosis caused by a recurrent activating R531Q mutation in the gamma 2-subunit of AMP-activated protein kinase (PRKAG2), not by phosphorylase kinase deficiency. *Am J Hum Genet.*2005; 76:1034–1049.
22. Steenhout P, Elmer C, Clercx A, Blum D, Gnat D, van Erum S et al. Carnitine deficiency with cardiomyopathy presenting as neonatal hydrops: successful response to carnitine therapy. *J Inherit Metab Dis.*1990; 13:69–75.
23. Hecher K, Snijders R, Campbell S, Nicolaides K. Fetal venous, intracardiac, and arterial blood flow measurements in intrauterine growth retardation: relationship with fetal blood gases. *Am J Obstet Gynecol.* 1995;173:10–15.
24. Kirkinen P, Jouppila P, Eik-Nes S. Umbilical vein blood flow in rhesus-isoimmunization. *Br J Obstet Gynaecol.*1983; 90:640–643.
25. Ruma MS, Moise KJ, Jr., Kim E, Murtha AP, Prutsman WJ, Hassan SS et al. Combined plasmapheresis and intravenous immune globulin for the treatment of severe maternal red cell alloimmunization. *Am J Obstet Gynecol.*2007; 196:138–136.
26. Rychik J, Tian Z, Bebbington M, Xu F, McCann M, Mann S, Wilson RD, Johnson MP. The twin-twin transfusion syndrome: spectrum of cardiovascular abnormality and development of a cardiovascular score to assess severity of disease. *Am J Obstet Gynecol.* 2007;197:392.e1–e8.
26. Albert TJ, Landon MB, Wheller JJ, Samuels P, Cheng RF, Gabbe S. Prenatal detection of fetal anomalies in pregnancies complicated by insulin-dependent diabetes mellitus. *Am J Obstet Gynecol.*1996;174: 1424–1428.
27. Rosenn B, Miodovnik M, Combs CA, Khoury J, Siddiqi TA. Glycemic thresholds for spontaneous abortion and congenital malformations in insulin-dependent diabetes mellitus. *Obstet Gynecol.*1994;84: 515–520.
28. Becerra JE, Khoury MJ, Cordero JF, Erickson JD. Diabetes mellitus during pregnancy and the risks for specific birth defects: a population-based case-control study. *Pediatrics.* 1990;85:1–9.
29. Meyer-Wittkopf M, Simpson JM, Sharland GK. Incidence of congenital heart defects in fetuses of diabetic mothers: a retrospective study of 326 cases. *Ultrasound Obstet Gynecol.* 1996;8:8–10.
30. Tyrala EE. The infant of the diabetic mother. *Obstet Gynecol Clin North Am.* 1996;23: 221–241.
31. Jaeggi ET, Fouron JC, Proulx F. Fetal cardiac performance in uncomplicated and well-controlled maternal type I diabetes. *Ultrasound Obstet Gynecol.*2001; 17:311–315.
32. Bergmans MG, Jonker GJ, Kock HC. Fetal supraventricular tachycardia. Review of the literature. *Obstet Gynecol Surv.*1985; 40:61–68.
33. Krapp M, Kohl T, Simpson JM, Sharland GK, Katalinic A, Gembruch U. Review of diagnosis, treatment, and outcome of fetal atrial flutter compared with supraventricular tachycardia. *Heart.*2003;89:913–917.
34. Simpson JM, Sharland GK. Fetal tachycardias: management and outcome of 127 consecutive cases. *Heart.*1998; 79:576–581.
35. Oudijk MA, Ruskamp JM, Ververs FF, Ambachtsheer EB, Stoutenbeek P, Visser GH et al. Treatment of fetal tachycardia with sotalol: transplacental pharmacokinetics and pharmacodynamics. *J Am Coll Cardiol.*2003; 42:765–770.
36. Jouannic JM, Delahaye S, Fermont L, Le Bidois J, Villain E, Dumez Y et al. Fetal supraventricular tachycardia: a role for amiodarone as second-line therapy? *Prenat Diagn.* 2003;23:152–156.
37. Ebenroth ES, Cordes TM, Darragh RK. Second-line treatment of fetal supraventricular tachycardia using flecainide acetate. *Pediatr Cardiol.*2001; 22:483–487.

38. Krapp M, Baschat AA, Gembruch U, Geipel A, Germer U. Flecainide in the intrauterine treatment of fetal supraventricular tachycardia. *Ultrasound Obstet Gynecol.*2002; 19:158–164.
39. Kohl T, Tercanli S, Kececioglu D, Holzgreve W. Direct fetal administration of adenosine for the termination of incessant supraventricular tachycardia. *Obstet Gynecol.*1995; 85:873–874.
40. Brucato A, Doria A, Frassi M, Castellino G, Franceschini F, Faden D et al. Pregnancy outcome in 100 women with autoimmune diseases and anti-Ro/SSA antibodies: a prospective controlled study. *Lupus.*2002; 11:716–721.
41. Menendez T, Achenbach S, Beinder E, Hofbeck M, Klinghammer L, Singer H et al. Usefulness of magnetocardiography for the investigation of fetal arrhythmias. *Am J Cardiol.* 2001;88:334–336.
42. Taylor MJ, Smith MJ, Thomas M, Green AR, Cheng F, Oseku-Afful S et al. Non-invasive fetal electrocardiography in singleton and multiple pregnancies. *BJOG.*2003; 110:668–678.
43. Groves AM, Allan LD, Rosenthal E. Outcome of isolated congenital complete heart block diagnosed in utero. *Heart.*1996; 75:190–194.
44. Jaeggi ET, Hamilton RM, Silverman ED, Zamora SA, Hornberger LK. Outcome of children with fetal, neonatal or childhood diagnosis of isolated congenital atrioventricular block. A single institution's experience of 30 years. *J Am Coll Cardiol.*2002; 39:130–137.
45. Saleeb S, Copel J, Friedman D, Buyon JP. Comparison of treatment with fluorinated glucocorticoids to the natural history of autoantibody-associated congenital heart block: retrospective review of the research registry for neonatal lupus. *Arthritis Rheum.*1999; 42:2335–2345.

Unique Aspects of Heart Failure in the Neonate

2

Jack F. Price

2.1 Introduction

Neonatal heart failure is characterized by many unique anatomic and physiologic features. Structural and functional differences between the mature and immature myocardium, as well as different etiologies of neonatal heart failure, pose challenges for the clinician when evaluating and treating the clinical syndrome of heart failure. Anatomically, the newborn myocardium is disorganized in its structure and has a lower density of contractile proteins. These features, as well as decreased cellular transport, may play a role in the relatively impaired contractile and relaxation functions of the immature heart. Despite these differences, the Frank-Starling relationship in the neonatal heart is intact and functional as cardiac output can be augmented with increased ventricular filling, as well as higher heart rates and inotropy. The treatment of the clinical syndrome of heart failure depends, in part, on the underlying cause of heart failure. In the presence of depressed myocardial contractility, unloading the myocardium with diuretics and afterload reducing agents often leads to symptomatic relief and improved cardiac output. Understanding the developmental changes in myocardial structure and function will add to the clinician's ability to provide optimal care of the newborn in the setting of a failing myocardium. The purpose of this chapter is to review the key differences between the neonatal heart failure and heart failure in the older child and adult.

2.2 Neonatal Cardiovascular Physiology

2.2.1 Post-natal Circulation

The fetal circulation undergoes dramatic changes at birth. Multiple physiologic transitions occur immediately in the newborn period and continue for the next several weeks. At delivery, more precisely when the umbilical cord and placenta are divided, the systemic

J.F.Pric e
TexasC hildren'sH ospital, BaylorC ollegeof M edicine, Houston,T X

R.E. Shaddy (ed.), *Heart Failure in Congenital Heart Disease*,
DOI: 10.1007/978-1-84996-480-7_2, © Springer-Verlag London Limited 2011

vascular resistance rises acutely. Concomitantly, the pulmonary vascular resistance begins to decrease. With this change in vascular resistance a series of other transitions occur. At the level of the ductus arteriosus, blood flow shifts from a fetal right-to-left circulation to a post-natal left-to-right shunt. Functionally, this usually occurs within 12 h of birth in term infants and may occur later in pre-term infants, leading to pulmonary overcirculation.[1] An increase in the partial pressure of oxygen in the blood acts as a stimulus for closure of the patent ductus arteriosus.[2,3] Additional factors that may play a role in ductal closure include nitric oxide and bradykinins.[4,5] Shortly after birth the ductus venosus also closes. It is speculated that decreased umbilical-placental blood flow to the ductus venosus leads to contraction of the vessel. Constriction of a sphincter at the origin of the ductus venosus may also contribute to closure.[6] Inhibitors of prostaglandin synthesis (indomethacin) have been shown to cause constriction of the ductus venosus in the fetal lamb.[7] The closure of the foramen ovale is caused by the passive forces of increased blood return to the left heart. In the fetus, a high pulmonary vascular resistance limits blood flow to the lungs. Less than 10% of the combined venous return enters the left atrium by way of the pulmonary veins. After birth, as the pulmonary vascular resistance falls and shunting in the ductus arteriosus becomes left-to-right, blood flow to the left atrium through the pulmonary veins increases substantially. Left atrial pressure rises and the septum primum apposes the crista, resulting in closure of the foramen ovale.

Pulmonary vascular resistance is high in the fetal lung but falls abruptly at birth (Fig. 2.1).[8]This rapid drop in pulmonary vascular resistance can be attributed to changes in both

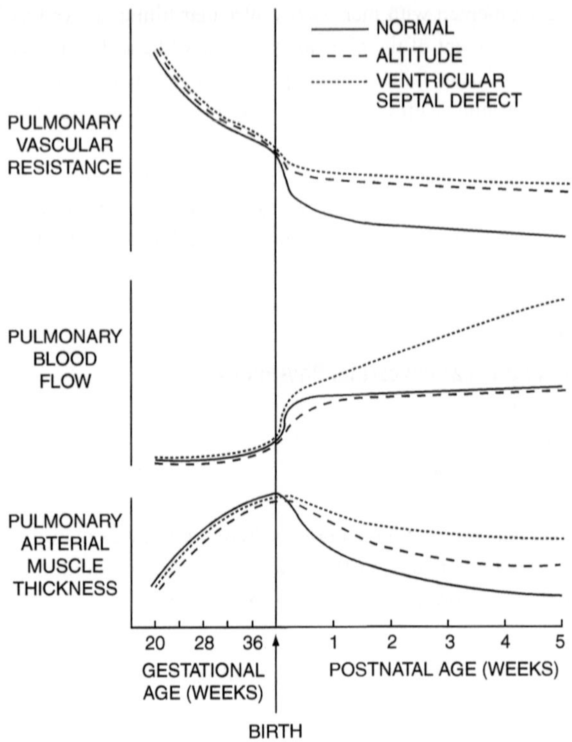

Fig.2. 1 Transitionsin f etal and neonatal hemodynamics. As pulmonary vascular resistance falls immediately at delivery and during the first few weeks of life, pulmonary blood flow increases and pulmonary arterial muscle thickness decreases (From[8] with permission)

ventilation and oxygenation.[9,10] Although ventilation is the major component of the fall of pulmonary vascular resistance, improved oxygenation also plays a role. Increases in oxygen concentration causes a modest increase in pulmonary blood flow and decrease in mean pulmonary artery pressure.[10] This may be partly due to the fact that oxygen modulates the production of the vasoactive substances nitric oxide and prostacyclin.

2.2.2 Neonatal Myocardium

At birth, physiologic changes in pressure and volume loads on the heart require that the neonatal myocardium compensate rapidly. Left ventricular volume and mass increase in early post-natal life in response to the changes in workloads of the left and right ventricles.[11,12] Myocyte numbers increase during this transition period. This hyperplastic growth response may be modulated by locally released ventricular acidic fibroblast growth factor.[13] Because of the increased demands of a higher vascular resistance to which it is exposed, myocyte proliferation occurs more rapidly in the left ventricle than the right. Cell growth continues through the first several weeks or months of life but becomes senescent later in life.[14] After these first few weeks, myocycte hypertrophy accounts for most of the increase in ventricular mass that occurs after birth. The post-natal hypertrophic growth response is thought to be stimulated by a change in workload demands on the ventricles as well as circulating growth factors and catecholamines. Acidic fibroblast growth factor and transforming growth factors produced by the cardiac myocycte may mediate cellular proliferation and differentiation.[15] Rising concentrations of circulating catecholamines also stimulate hypertrophy of cultured neonatal myocytes.[16]

The neonatal myocycte is quite different structurally from the mature myocyte. The immature cardiac myocyte is rounded, relatively short, and quite disorganized intracellularly (Fig. 2.2). It changes into a slender and longer shape and takes on a more organized ultrastructural appearance as it matures. The myofibrils are contractile proteins that help to give the myocyte its shape and structural organization. In the mature cell the myofibrils are densely concentrated and are aligned in parallel with the axis of the cell, organized into alternating rows of mitochondria. In the neonatal cardiomyocyte, however, the myofibrils are relatively less dense and are more likely to be situated along the periphery of the cell (Fig. 2.3). The more central portion of the myocyte is made up of disorganized clumps of mitochondria and nuclei.[11,17,18] The mitochondria increase in number, relative volume, and cristae thickness as the cell matures.[19,20] These changes occur in concert with postnatal developmental changes in substrate metabolism. As the mitochondria increase in volume and take on a more orderly relationship, the myocardium matures to utilize activated long chain fatty acids as its primary source of energy rather than carbohydrate.[21–23]

The sarcomere is the contractile unit of cardiac muscle and is organized into overlapping strands of thick and think filaments (contractile proteins). The number of sarcomeres increases and their organizational structure is transformed during the first few months of life.[14] During development, several different isoforms of contractile proteins change their expression, and therefore the functional properties of the sarcomere.[24]

The cardiac myocyte plasma membrane, or sarcolemma, is made up of ion channels and pumps that allow for transsarcolemmal transport of calcium and other ions. It is recognized

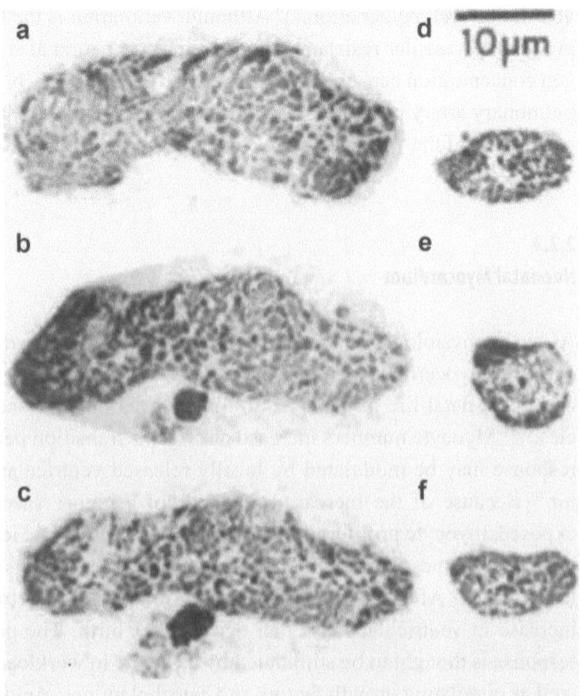

Fig. 2. 2 Crosss ectionsf rom adult (**a**–**c**) and neonatal myocytes (**d**–**f**). There are significant differences in size and shape between the adult and immature cells (From[17] withpe rmission)

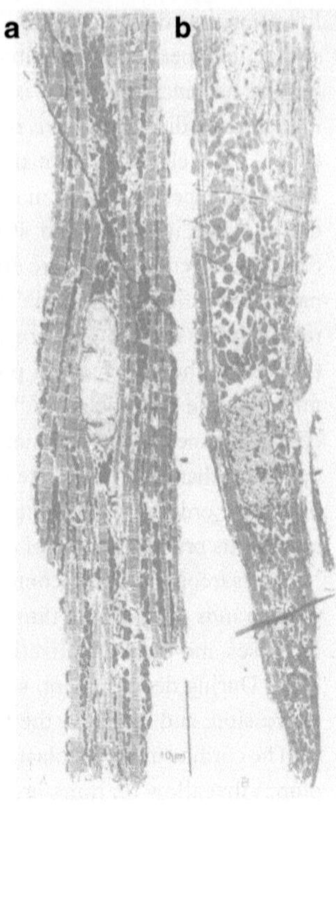

Fig. 2. 3 Longitudinal sections from adult (**a**) and neonatal (**b**) myocytes. The neonatal myocyte is less organized and contains fewer contractile elements. Unlike the adult, alternating rows of mitochondria and myofibrils are not present in the immature myocyte (From[17]w ithpe rmission)

that the immature heart is more dependent on extracellular calcium for myocardial contraction. Age-dependent density and current properties of ion channels may impact on myocardial performance. In human atria, decreased calcium current density has been demonstrated in children when compared to adults.[25] Calcium ion current in the atria also inactivates more rapidly in infants and children compared to adults.[26] The sarcolemma is tightly associated with the sarcoplasmic reticulum, a tubular meshwork surrounding the myofibrils and responsible for the uptake and release of cytosolic calcium. The sarcoplasmic reticulum from fetal sheep contains a lower density of Ca^{2+} channels and decreased pump activity compared to maternal sheep.[27] These differences in composition and function of calcium transporters may contribute to decreased myocardial reserve and contractility in the immature myocardium.

The extracellular matrix represents another unique feature of the neonatal myocardium. This complex of proteoglycans, glycoproteins, and collagen provides structural support and contributes to the active and passive properties of the myocyte.[28] The composition of the extracellular matrix changes over time. Laminin, a matrix protein found in the basal laminae and important for cell adhesion, is sparsely distributed in the embryonic myocardium and localized to discrete areas of the matrix related to the sarcolemma during fetal development.[29–31] Only later, in the mature myocyte, is laminin found throughout the basement membrane, closely associated with the Z discs of the sarcomere.[63] This association suggests a possible mechanical contribution of the extracellular matrix to myocardial contraction and relaxation.[28]

2.3 Ventricular Contraction and Relaxation

During the first few weeks and months of life, the composition of the myocardium changes significantly and with that the functional capacity of the heart. The immature myocardium is less compliant, generates less contractile force and is inefficiently shaped when compared to the mature heart. Developmental changes in the composition of the sarcolemma, contractile proteins, mitochondria and extracellular matrix play important roles in the myocyte's ability to develop sarcomeric shortening and myocardial tension. A combination of a greater ratio of noncontractile elements to contractile elements in the neonatal heart and less organized and efficient myofibrils impact on myocardial contractility.[32] The neonatal heart is not capable of generating the same tension per unit cross-sectional area as the myocardium of adults. Numerous studies have demonstrated developmental differences in myocardial contractility.[33–37] Friedman et al. showed that the active tension generated in fetal lamb cardiac muscle is significantly reduced compared to adult lambs (Fig. 2.4).[38] Fetal myocardial contractility is reduced at all cardiac muscle lengths. Additionally, at any given tension, the velocity of shortening is diminished compared to the adult. The resting, or passive tension, is also higher in the fetus than the adult suggesting reduced compliance of these muscles.

Despite a relatively reduced ability to develop tension, the neonatal myocardial contractility can be augmented with inotropes. Anderson et al. demonstrated that an infusion

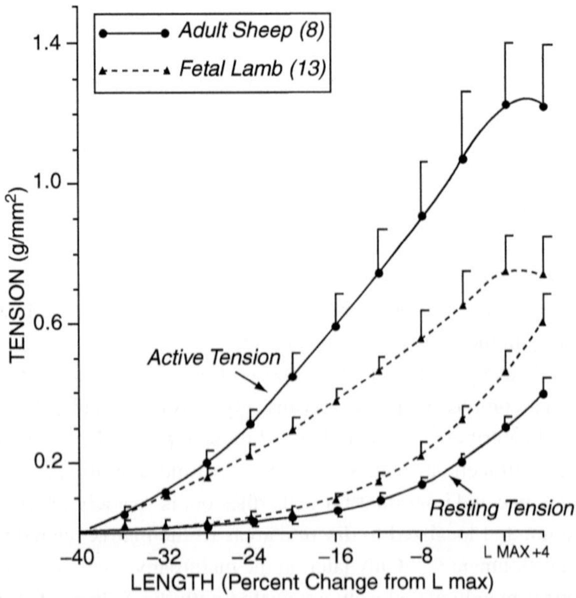

Fig. 2.4 Isometricpa ssivea nd active length-tension curves from the fetal lamb and adult sheep. At all muscle lengths, the active tension generated by fetal cardiac muscle is less than that of the adult. Passive tension is higher in the fetus than the adult, consistent with diminished compliance(From[38]w ith permission)

of isoproterenol in fetal and neonatal lambs can enhance percentage systolic fractional shortening and the rate of rise of left ventricular pressure even before the chronotropic effects of the drug take effect.[39] Additionally, the myocardial contractility was more enhanced in the neonatal lamb than the fetal lamb. Park et al. confirmed the developmental changes in myocardial contractility in dogs when exposed to isoproterenol and further showed a sensitivity to calcium in the newborn that was absent in the adult.[37] When calcium was added to cardiac muscle, active tension and the maximum rate of contraction markedly increased in newborn dogs but not in adult dogs. Altered sarcoplasmic reticulum function and sensitivity of the myofilaments to calcium in the immature myocardium are possible reasons for this difference.

Although the neonatal myocardium has the capacity to augment contractility when exposed to inotropic agents, that capacity may be reduced compared to the older infant and child.[40] Higher baseline concentrations of catecholamines may limit the ability of the immature myocyte to further increase cardiac output. Circulating concentrations of norepinephrine are elevated at birth[41] and may cause a transient increase in myocardial contractility in the perinatal period. Pressure loads on the immature myocardium can also negatively impact on cardiac function. The fetal myocardium is very sensitive to afterload and has a limited capacity for improved cardiac performance in the presence of raised arterial pressure.[42] This limited capacity for improved function and high baseline levels of circulating catecholamines suggest that cardiac performance is normally near maximum in the fetus. Even so, cardiac output can be augmented to some degree with various manipulations including volume loading and catecholamines.

The increase in pressure and volume that occurs as blood enters the heart is determined by the compliance of the ventricular myocardium. The compliance of the newborn heart is relatively reduced compared to the adult. Ventricular filling is affected by several factors including the active and passive properties of myocardium, ventricular interdependence, and the pericardium. Developmental changes in the extracellular matrix and cytoskeleton as well as the decreased ability of the neonatal myocardium to sequester calcium from the cytosol[43] may also impact on the mechanical relaxation properties of the neonatal heart.

The newborn myocardium responds to volume loading differently than the adult myocardium. In the immature canine heart (3–4 weeks of age), left ventricular filling volume is reduced at pressures greater than 5 mmHg when compared to adult canine myocardium (Fig. 2.5). The immature heart is stiffer and requires a smaller relative volume to achieve a given filling pressure.[44] Additionally, midwall sarcomere length is substantially shorter at higher pressures in the left ventricle of the immature canine than the mature canine.[44] Further evidence of diminished ventricular compliance is supported by studies in immature lambs. The pressure-volume and wall tension relationships of the left and right ventricles are similar in the fetal lamb but are significantly different in the newborn period and in adult sheep. Higher pressures are achieved with a given volume load in the right ventricle compared to the left. In the neonate, left ventricular compliance is altered and becomes intermediate to that of the fetus and adult. At all ages the right ventricle is more compliant than the left (Fig. 2.6)[45]. The influence of ventricular interdependence also differs by age, with filling of one ventricle reducing the distensibility of the opposite ventricle, occurring most profoundly in the fetus and less so in the adult myocardium (Fig. 2.7). Ventricular compliance increases with maturation throughout many species.[33,38,46–49]

The Frank-Starling curve is operative and effective in the neonatal heart although shifted due to a limited capacity for developing active tension. Augmenting preload within the normal physiologic range of 2–8 mmHg in fetal lambs is associated with augmented left ventricular shortening and stroke volume (Fig. 2.8).[50] When volume loaded to left ventricular end-diastolic pressures greater than 8 mmHg, however, very little further increase in shortening is achieved. Compared to more mature myocardium, little change in cardiac output is seen when the immature ventricle is volume loaded.[51]

This limited capacity for augmenting cardiac output with ventricular filling means that increasing heart rate becomes an important mechanism for increasing cardiac output in the neonate.[52] Naturally occurring heart rate changes associated with changes in venous return to the heart combine to produce a positive relationship between heart rate and left

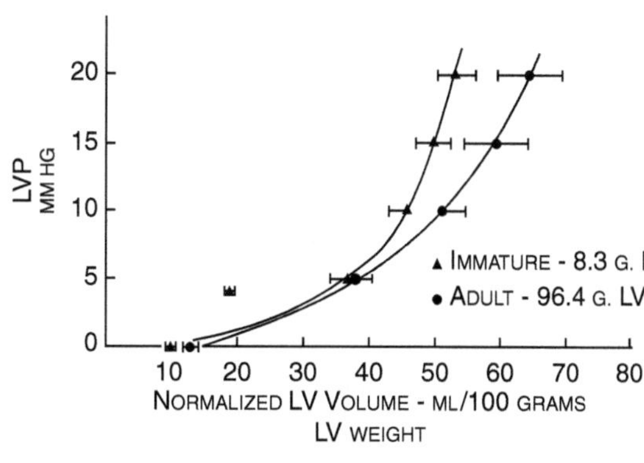

Fig. 2.5 Mean pressure-normalized volume curves for the immature and adult dog. Left ventricular pressures (LVP) are greater for normalized left ventricular volume in the immature dog compared to the adult (decreased compliance) and the curves diverge at pressures greater than 5 mmHg (From[44] with permission)

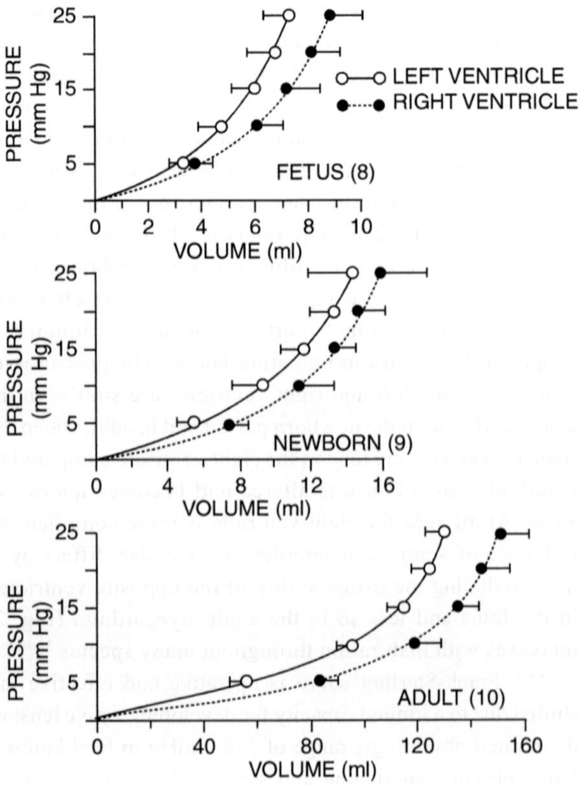

Fig. 2.6 Meanpre ssure-volume curves for the fetal, newborn, and adult heart. Horizontal bars represent ± standard error. Fetal left and right ventricles were not significantly different. In the newborn and adult, relatively greater LV stiffness was observed with shift of the pressure–volume curves to the left of the RV curve[45]

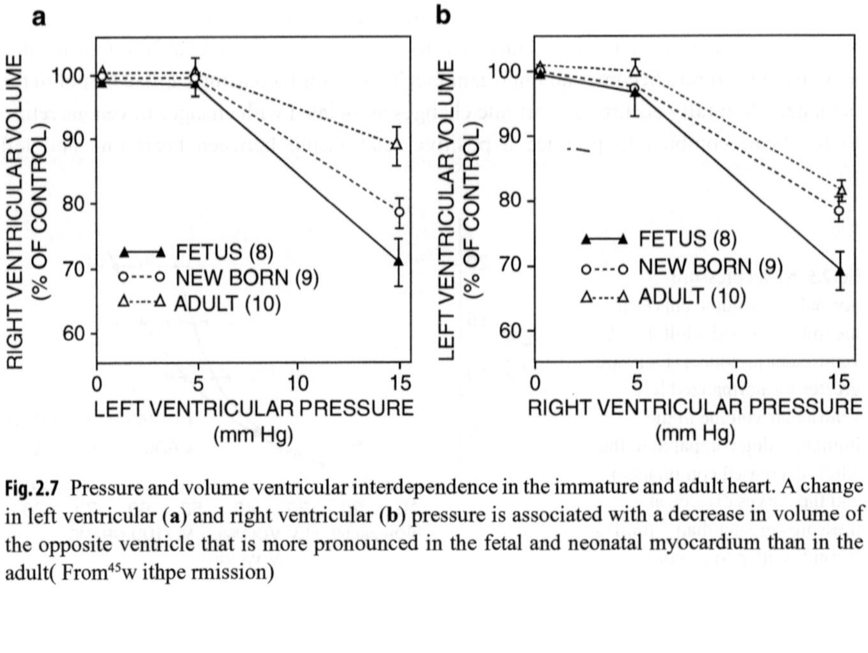

Fig. 2.7 Pressure and volume ventricular interdependence in the immature and adult heart. A change in left ventricular (**a**) and right ventricular (**b**) pressure is associated with a decrease in volume of the opposite ventricle that is more pronounced in the fetal and neonatal myocardium than in the adult(From[45]w ithpe rmission)

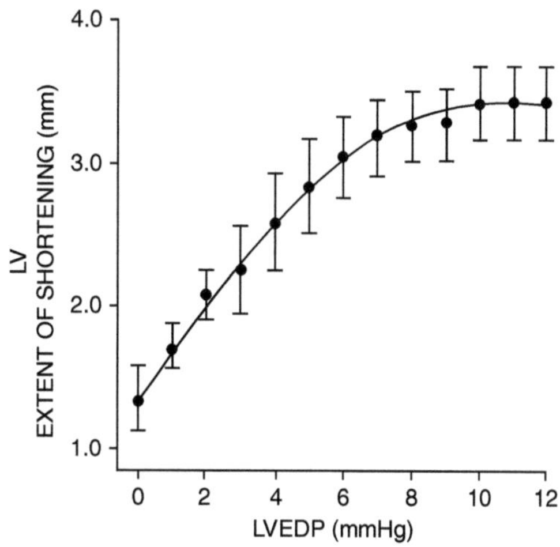

Fig. 2.8 The influence of left ventricular end-diastolic pressure (LVEDP) on left ventricular shortening. In fetal lambs, increased LVEDP (2.5–8 mmHg) was associated with a 68% change in LV shortening. There was no further increase in ventricular shortening beyond an LVEDP of 10 mmHg. Each point and vertical bars represent mean ±SE (From[50] with permission)

ventricular output.[53] The increase in ventricular output observed at higher heart rates is likely not solely a chronotropic phenomena in a stiff heart. Anderson et al. showed that an increase in heart rate in the fetal lamb is associated with an increase in the maximum rate of rise of left ventricular pressure and fractional shortening.[39]

2.4 Sympathetic Activity

The sympathetic nervous system is the chief regulator of the neurohormonal response of heart failure. Afferent baroreceptor input to the brain signals low cardiac output states. Efferent sympathetic pathways are then activated, causing vasoconstriction of the renal and peripheral vasculature as well as the release of renin and angiotensin II and the non-osmotic release of arginine vasopressin. As mentioned previously, baseline plasma concentrations of catecholamines are elevated in the neonate compared to the older child and adult.[41,54] A high resting adrenergic state is thought to be at least partly responsible for a limited reserve in contractility in newborn lambs that improves with age.[40] Myocardial catecholamine concentrations, however, are higher in the adult than the fetus and neonate.[55] Several studies have demonstrated that cardiac sympathetic innervation is incomplete in the neonate but gradually matures postnatally.[38,54–56] In dogs, the functional significance of this difference is an inability to maintain significant cardiac functional responses after repeated sympathetic stimulation in the immature myocardium and that adrenal integrity, therefore, is necessary for appropriate cardiac output response to sympathetic stimulation.[57]

Developmental differences in the hemodynamic response to similar doses of exogenous catecholamines exists and is likely due in large part to differences in drug pharmacokinetics between the age groups.[58] Researchers have demonstrated age-dependent differences in the clearance rates of sympathomimetic inotropes.[59,60] Dopamine clearance rates decrease significantly with age, with rates in children under 2 years of age nearly twice as great as older children. Because they have a higher percentage of body water than adults, neonates and infants have a larger volume of distribution for water soluble drugs, including phosphodiesterase inhibitors[61,62] and digoxin.[63] Individual differences also affect clearance rates, including factors such as hypoperfusion to vital organs, systemic inflammatory response syndrome, and differences in enzyme activity.[58,64]

Age-related variation in the hemodynamic response to exogenous catecholamines may also result from different responses to the adrenergic receptor. While the relative receptor density of β-adrenergic receptor subtypes is similar in both neonatal and adult rats, a difference in response to receptor stimulation can be measured.[65] At low agonist concentrations, β_2-adrenergic receptor activation improves contractile performance in the neonatal rat but has no effect on the adult rat myocardium. The efficiency of β-adrenergic signal transduction is further affected by the relatively low concentration of the inhibitory (G_i) G protein isoform in the neonatal rat ventricular myocardium.[66] Moreover, developmentally controlled enhancement of phospholambin and troponin I phosphorylation may contribute to cAMP-mediated relaxation.

Prolonged stimulation of the β-adrenergic receptor normally leads to desensitization and down-regulation. The neonate is unique, however, in that desensitization does not occur with chronic stimulation of the agonist-occupied receptor. In fact, the opposite occurs – the receptor becomes sensitized and the response to stimulation is enhanced.[67]I n the rat, this agonist-induced sensitization is thought to occur as a result of increased expression of adenylyl cyclase[68] coupled with altered G protein function[68–70] It is not known if a lack of desensitization or enhanced adrenergic response occurs similarly in humans.

2.5 Etiology of Heart Failure

Neonatal heart failure can manifest in both acquired and congenital forms with etiologies as disparate as structural, metabolic and environmental in origin. Following are features of some of the more common causes of heart failure in the neonatal period.

2.5.1 Excessive Pulmonary Blood Flow

Some might not consider symptomatic pulmonary overcirculation to be a true form of heart failure. After all, ventricular systolic function is usually preserved or even hyperdynamic in lesions associated with a large net left-to-right shunt and low cardiac output is not a typical finding in this situation. But if heart failure is a clinical syndrome characterized by elevated filling pressures, compensatory activation of the neurohormonal system and progressive symptomatology, then pulmonary overcirculation certainly deserves to be recognized as a form of heart failure.

As in heart failure due to left ventricular dysfunction, circulatory adaptive mechanisms are triggered in symptomatic pulmonary overcirculation to preserve cardiac output and end organ perfusion. The sympathetic nervous system is activated and plasma concentrations of norepinephrine increase, stimulating the renin–angiotensin–aldosterone system, causing peripheral vasoconstriction and increased heart rate. Plasma norepinephrine levels are elevated in infants and children with heart failure due to left-to-right shunting lesions,[71] and these concentrations normalize after surgical repair of the structural defects.[72] Likewise, plasma concentrations of arginine vasopressin, a neurohormone that causes peripheral vasoconstriction and free water retention, are also increased in children with heart failure due to shunting lesions as well as in situations of ventricular dysfunction.[73] Natriuretic peptides are secreted by the atria and ventricles in response to myocardial stretch due to pressure or volume loads on the heart. Plasma levels of atrial natriuretic peptide,[74] and B-type natriuretic peptide,[75] are elevated in children with congenital heart disease and correlate with Qp:Qs in patients with left-to-right intracardiac shunts.

In acyanotic cardiac lesions such as ventricular septal defect and complete atrioventricular canal defect, signs and symptoms of heart failure usually develop during the neonatal period, as the pulmonary vascular resistance falls. Signs such as tachypnea, retractions, grunting and diaphoresis with feeding usually herald this change in physiology. Other acyanotic lesions also associated with large left-to-right shunting include the patent ductus arteriosus, aortopulmonary window and systemic arteriovenous malformations. These typical "run off" lesions may manifest with signs of heart failure in the first few days (in premature infants) or weeks of life with bounding pulses in addition to signs of respiratory compromise. If left uncorrected, these defects can lead to pulmonary vascular disease over time.

Cyanotic cardiac defects can also be associated with pulmonary overcirculation and heart failure and include truncus arteriosus, total anomalous pulmonary venous connection, tricuspid atresia (without obstructed pulmonary blood flow) and double outlet right ventricle (without obstructed pulmonary blood flow). In these lesions, an admixture of highly oxygen-saturated and less oxygen-saturated blood occurs at the atrial, ventricular or great arterial level and the mixed blood is then sent to the pulmonary and systemic circulations, taking the path of least resistance. Chest radiography may reveal increased pulmonary vascular markings despite low systemic arterial oxygen saturations. Classic signs of heart failure are also seen in infants with unrepaired or non-palliated forms of cyanotic pulmonary overcirculation and include cardiomegaly, hepatomegaly, tachypnea and poor weight gain.

Children born with ductal-dependent systemic blood flow lesions such as hypoplastic left heart syndrome or a variant thereof can develop signs of heart failure while being administered prostaglandin E1 and awaiting surgical palliation. As pulmonary vascular resistance falls, increased pulmonary blood flow may lead to heart failure of pulmonary overcirculation and low cardiac output syndrome. This progressive imbalance of Qp:Qs places an increased demand on the systemic right ventricle to maintain cardiac output while producing a falsely reassuring high systemic oxygen saturation. These newborns may develop pulmonary vascular congestion, poor perfusion, metabolic acidosis and end-organ injury from inadequate systemic blood flow. Efforts to limit excessive pulmonary blood flow and increase pulmonary vascular resistance by either reducing alveolar PO2 or increasing alveolar PCO2 may improve cardiac output. Strategies such as intubation and administration of inspired CO2,[76,77] reduction of minute ventilation, and adding nitrogen to the inspired gases to create a subambient FiO2 concentration have been employed with variable success. Once a patient has been stabilized and acidosis has been corrected a more definitive therapy such as the Norwood procedure or Sano modification of stage 1 reconstruction is required.

2.5.2 Pressure Overload

Some forms of congenital heart disease can manifest with signs of heart failure in the early newborn period (first 3 days of life). Infants with critical aortic or pulmonary valvar stenosis may present with shock or cyanosis, respectively. Critical coarctation of the aorta or interrupted aortic arch may also present in the first few days of life as the ductus arteriosus closes. These left-sided obstructive lesions often coexist, and the clinical spectrum can vary between an isolated bicuspid aortic valve with minimal obstruction to hypoplastic left heart syndrome. The right ventricle generally will support the systemic circulation in the setting of a widely patent ductus arteriosus. When the ductus closes, however, the right ventricle cannot adequately perfuse the systemic circulation resulting in a profound metabolic acidosis, and if untreated, multiorgan system failure and death. Initial stabilization of neonates with low cardiac output and hypotension with suspected heart disease may require volume resuscitation, correction of acidosis and initiation of inotropic support. Until a diagnosis can be determined, an infusion of prostaglandin E1 should be started in an effort to maintain patency of the ductus arteriosus. Opening the ductus provides palliative blood flow to the systemic circulation in the presence of critical left-sided obstructive lesions such as critical aortic stenosis, coarctation, interrupted aortic arch, and hypoplastic left heart syndrome and allows for augmented pulmonary blood flow in the situation of critical pulmonary stenosis. The benefits of prostaglandin E1 in these clinical scenarios usually outweigh any risks or side effects (e.g. apnea, fever, peripheral vasodilation). If the patient is anemic, transfusion with packed red blood cells can improve oxygen delivery. Concurrent with starting prostaglandin should be intubation and control of ventilation as a key element of decreasing metabolic demand. Additionally, positive pressure ventilation can improve left ventricular dysfunction by decreasing left ventricular afterload.[78]

Once the patient has been stabilized and a diagnosis confirmed, a more definitive intervention can be performed. In valvar aortic stenosis, the leaflets are usually dysplastic, thickened, doming in systole and the aortic valve is frequently bicommissural. Balloon valvuloplasty for either critical pulmonary or aortic valve stenosis can provide rapid hemodynamic relief. Balloon valvuloplasty may be the treatment of choice for infants with aortic stenosis and depressed left ventricular systolic function, avoiding surgical intervention in the newborn period. Results of balloon valvuloplasty are comparable to surgical valvotomy and the treatment of choice usually depends on institutional experience and preference. Balloon valvuloplasty has been associated with decreased residual gradient, higher degree of aortic insufficiency, and an increased need or reintervention as compared with surgical valvotomy.[79] Surgical repair of coarctation of the aorta or aortic arch hypoplasia is the preferred treatment for native coarctation of the aorta in the newborn period.

Ventricular dysfunction caused by systemic hypertension can also lead to heart failure. Although rare in children, systemic hypertension is thought to be the etiology of dilated cardiomyopathy with depressed myocardial function in pediatric patients with neuroblastoma and Wilms tumor. In neuroblastoma, high levels of circulating catecholamines cause peripheral vasoconstriction and raise the systemic vascular resistance. Additionally, norepinephrine is directly toxic to the myocardium and a protracted period of high concentrations can lead to myocyte drop out and apoptosis. Patients with Wilms tumor may have high circulating levels of renin which also increases systemic vascular resistance. Treatment of these tumors can lead to reverse remodeling of the myocardium and improved ventricular function. Other renal causes of systemic hypertension (e.g. renal artery stenosis, nephritis) in children may also lead to ventricular dysfunction and heart failure, but these diseases often manifest with ventricular hypertrophy initially.

2.5.3 Valvular Insufficiency

Pulmonary valvar insufficiency causing ventricular dysfunction or heart failure is usually a result of previous surgery or catheter-based interventions on the pulmonary valve. Congenital forms of pulmonary insufficiency are also recognized, such as absent pulmonary valve syndrome.

Tricuspid regurgitation is an uncommon cause of heart failure in children. Clinically significant tricuspid regurgitation is most often seen in patients with Ebstein's anomaly, a congenital defect of the heart in which the annular attachments of the tricuspid valve are displaced towards the apex of the right ventricle. The ventricle becomes divided into an "atrialized" inlet portion and functional apical and infundibular portions. The tricuspid valve leaflets fail to coapt, causing severe tricuspid regurgitation and right atrial enlargement. Prograde pulmonary blood flow may be significantly compromised and right ventricular function may eventually deteriorate. Symptomatic patients diagnosed in the newborn or infant period usually have the most severe form of the disease and develop signs of heart failure early on. The mortality rate is high among patients who require surgical intervention at this age. Older individuals with less severe disease may develop symptoms of right heart failure including hepatomegaly, jugular venous distention, peripheral edema and dyspnea with exertion. Atrial arrhythmias are also common in this cohort. Other causes of significant tricuspid regurgitation include endocarditis and tricuspid valvar dysplasia.

While tricuspid regurgitation may result in a dilated and poorly functioning right ventricle, the reverse is also true. Functional tricuspid regurgitation, in the setting of a structurally normal valve, may occur secondary to pressure or volume loads on the right ventricle. A hypertensive right ventricle will eventually dilate, causing the annulus to stretch and the valve leaflets to fail to coapt properly resulting in tricuspid regurgitation. Elevated right ventricular pressures and subsequent valvar incompetence in the neonate are usually caused by persistent pulmonary hypertension, left atrial hypertension (e.g., mitral stenosis), or pulmonary valve stenosis. Correcting the underlying cause of right ventricular hypertension may reduce the degree of valvar regurgitation and ameliorate the clinical features of heart failure. A volume load on right ventricle can also lead to annular dilation and incompetence. Congenital defects such as total anomalous pulmonary venous return, cerebral or hepatic arteriovenous malformations, and absent pulmonary valve syndrome cause an increase in blood flow to the right heart producing progressive right ventricular dilation.

Other forms of valvar insufficiency causing heart failure in the newborn period are rare. Aortic insufficiency in the neonate usually occurs secondary to surgery or a catheter-based intervention. A dilated aortic root, as a result of neonatal Marfan syndrome, is frequently associated with aortic insufficiency and may cause left ventricular dilation and dysfunction.[80] The mitral valve may also be affected in Marfan syndrome, causing leaflet prolapse and regurgitation. Congenital mitral regurgitation leading to heart failure in the neonate is rare and is usually associated with other cardiac defects or occurs secondary to dilated cardiomyopathy or infarction of the papillary muscles.

2.5.4 Ischemic Cardiomyopathy

Myocardial ischemia, as a result of anomalous origin of the coronary arteries, is an infrequent and potentially reversible cause congestive heart failure in the neonate and infant. Anomalous origin of the left coronary artery from the pulmonary artery (ALCAPA) usually is an isolated malformation that occurs during embryogenesis. In the fetus, pulmonary artery pressure is relatively high and coronary artery perfusion is therefore adequate. Postnatally, however, as pulmonary vascular resistance falls, pulmonary arterial pressure decreases leading to diminished left coronary artery (LCA) perfusion. Blood flow to the left coronary artery is then dependent on retrograde filling from collateral vessels that originate from the higher pressure right coronary artery (RCA).[81] A small left-to-right shunt is created with oxygenated blood from the RCA coursing through collaterals to the LCA and ultimately draining into the pulmonary artery. This failure of antegrade perfusion through the LCA leads to myocardial ischemia that may cause subendocardial or transmural infarction and, eventually, the clinical syndrome of heart failure.

Most patients with ALCAPA develop signs of heart failure in the first few weeks or months of life. The earliest signs of heart failure include failure to thrive, tachypnea, wheezing, diaphoresis, and angina-like episodes that manifest as sudden inconsolability and pallor.[82] A gallop rhythm and blowing holosystolic murmur of mitral insufficiency may be appreciated on physical exam. Chest radiograph typically reveals cardiomegaly and prominent pulmonary vascular markings may be present. The electrocardiogram classically demonstrates ST segment elevation in the anterolateral leads and Q waves in leads I and aVL.

Although the signs and symptoms of heart failure in ALCAPA can be relieved with medicinal therapy, the goal should be to correct any hemodynamic derangements and stabilize the patient in preparation for surgery. Myocardial ischemia in ALCAPA is potentially reversible with surgical repair[83,84] and improved ventricular function is frequently observed after reimplantation of the coronary artery.[85]

2.6 Treatment of Heart Failure in the Neonate

Because the management of chronic heart failure is discussed in a separate chapter, this discussion will serve to highlight the unique features of treatment of the newborn with decompensated heart failure, in particular the neonate with heart failure secondary to ventricular dysfunction. The clinical spectrum of heart failure is broad in the newborn period, ranging from the hypoxemic infant with persistent pulmonary hypertension and fulminant right-sided heart failure to the hydropic infant with neonatal myocarditis and severely depressed left ventricular function, to the robust child with respiratory insufficiency caused by diastolic heart failure of hypertrophic cardiomyopathy. Clearly, the care of such patients must be individualized as one aims to provide symptomatic relief, correct metabolic abnormalities and reverse hemodynamic derangements. Achievement of these goals requires familiarity with the risks and benefits of particular therapies as well as knowledge of the pharmacokinetic differences between the neonate and older child. Treatment options for decompensated heart failure are limited and almost all are untested in children. Most of the data and insight relied upon for managing pediatric patients with advanced heart failure have been derived from studies and experience in adults, the majority of whom have an ischemic etiology for their LV dysfunction. Because there are no formal recommendations for the treatment of advanced heart failure in children, we must heed the findings of adult trials, reflect on reliable anecdotal experience and respect the principle that we should first do no harm.

Intravenous diuretics (usually loop diuretics) are considered standard of care therapy for the initial treatment of decompensated heart failure in neonates and children and should be given without delay. Diuretic "resistance" may respond to the addition of thiazide diuretics such as metolazone or intravenous chlorothiazide. Another consideration is the use of a continuous infusion of a loop diuretic instead of scheduled intermittent dosing when patients fail to respond to diuretic therapy. Fluid restriction in neonates is rarely ever necessary. During intravenous diuretic therapy the treating physician should frequently monitor for a variety of side effects including electrolyte disturbances, renal insufficiency and hypotension. Because of immature renal secretory control in the neonate, urinary loss of potassium, magnesium and calcium can be profound.

Newborns with decompensated heart failure and reduced blood pressure with normal or low systemic vascular resistance should be considered for inotropic therapy. In these patients, inotropic agents may be necessary to maintain circulatory function and improve end-organ function. Milrinone, sometimes referred to as an inodilator, is a phosphodiesterase inhibitor that acts by increasing cyclic adenosine monophosphate (cAMP), thereby providing inotropy with additional afterload reduction. Milrinone also reduces pulmonary vascular tone and is less likely to cause tachycardia like other inotropic agents. Although it can be proarrhythmic, milrinone is not typically associated with the sustained tachycardia, increased myocardial oxygen consumption or elevated systemic vascular resistance that often occurs with the use of other inotropic agents. Only a few studies have evaluated the safety and efficacy of milrinone for the treatment of decompensated heart failure in adults, and thus far they have failed to show any clinical benefit when used for this indication.[86,87] In fact, the data suggest that milrinone may actually increase the risk of arrhythmias and other morbidities. In the OPTIME trial, 949 adults hospitalized with an exacerbation of chronic heart failure were randomized to receive either a 48-h infusion of milrinone or placebo. The primary outcome measure was hospitalization for cardiac cause within 60 days of enrollment. There was no difference in the median number of cardiac-related hospital days between the milrinone group (6 days) and the placebo group (7 days, $p = 0.71$). More concerning was the incidence of adverse events associated with milrinone use. Sustained hypotension and atrial arrhythmias occurred significantly more frequently in patients receiving milrinone. The authors concluded that their results did not support the routine use of milrinone as an adjunct to standard therapy for the treatment of heart failure exacerbations.[88] A few studies have examined the cardiovascular effects of phosphodiesterase inhibitors in children.[89,90] In the PRIMACORP study, milrinone used in neonates in the immediate postoperative period reduced the risk of low cardiac output syndrome.[91] Dosing and utility of milrinone for the treatment of decompensated pediatric heart failure are not known. Previously, in adults, a bolus was given prior to starting a continuous infusion, but this is no longer thought to be necessary since after 2 h of infusion the hemodynamic effects are the same with or without bolus therapy. Infusions should be started at a relatively low dose (0.1–0.3 mcg/kg/min) and uptitrated to a maximum of approximately 0.75 mcg/kg/min, depending on systemic blood pressure response.

An alternative to milrinone, especially in situations of hypotension, are the sympathomimetic agents dobutamine, dopamine and epinephrine. These agents stimulate adrenergic receptors in the myocardium and smooth muscle causing increased cAMP concentrations and enhanced inotropy and vascular resistance. They may also result in tachycardia, increased myocardial oxygen consumption and an increased incidence of arrhythmias.

Dobutamine is a sympathomimetic drug that is commonly used in adults for the treatment of decompensated heart failure. It stimulates β-adrenergic receptors in the myocardium and peripheral vasculature causing increased myocardial contractility and decreased peripheral and pulmonary vascular tone.[92] Improved inotropy coupled with afterload reduction previously seemed like a desirable combination for patients with symptomatic heart failure but subsequent controlled studies have demonstrated significant adverse effects when dobutamine is used in this situation. Data from the Flolan International Randomized Survival Trial (FIRST) demonstrated a higher mortality rate among NYHA class III and IV heart failure patients who were treated with intravenous continuous dobutamine compared to those who were not (70.5 percent vs. 37.1 percent, $p = 0.0001$).[93] Dobutamine is also known to increase heart rate, myocardial oxygen consumption and the incidence of atrial and ventricular arrhythmias. No controlled studies have been performed in children assessing safety or efficacy of dobutamine for advanced heart failure. If dobutamine is to be used for the treatment of decompensated heart failure, it should be started at the lowest dose capable of achieving the desired effect and should be weaned or discontinued as soon as possible. Doses of 2.5–10 mcg/kg/min are capable of increasing cardiac output, reducing systemic vascular resistance and improving stroke volume. Higher doses are unlikely to provide further improvement in hemodynamics and are more likely to be associated with adverse effects.

Dopamine is a sympathomimetic that stimulates β-adrenergic receptors, as well as α-adrenergic receptors and dopaminergic receptors on the peripheral vasculature. It acts predominantly on β1 receptors in the myocardium causing increased contractility and heart rate at doses of 3 mcg/kg/min and greater. The α-adrenergic receptor response is seen at doses of 5 mcg/kg/min and higher, causing peripheral vasoconstriction and overwhelming any β2-induced vasodilation. The dopaminergic or renal effects occur at doses less than 3 mcg/kg/min, augmenting renal blood flow. Whether this improves renal function or urine output in patients with heart failure remains controversial. Dopamine is a good choice for patients in low cardiac output when sustained pressor support is needed quickly. Common side effects of dopamine infusions include tachycardia, ventricular arrhythmias, hypertension and headache.

In life-threatening situations or cardiogenic shock, an epinephrine infusion is indicated. Even low dose epinephrine boluses can sustain systemic pressure until a more reliable therapy can be initiated. Epinephrine stimulates both α and β receptors with pressor effects occurring at doses of 0.02 mcg/kg/min or greater. Although epinephrine may increase blood pressure, heart rate and contractility it also may cause ischemia, atrial or ventricular arrhythmias and increased myocardial oxygen consumption.

When catecholamine-resistant hypotension is encountered, a vasopressin infusion may improve systemic vascular resistance. Vasopressin has not been studied in a controlled fashion for this indication in heart failure patients, but at our institution we have used doses of 0.01–0.05 units/kg/h for the purpose of treating hypotension in end-stage heart failure. A calcium chloride infusion may also support blood pressure and provide increased contractility in emergency situations. We have typically used doses of 2.5–5.0 mg/kg/h, while monitoring ionized calcium concentrations.

2.7 Summary

The syndrome of heart failure in neonates differs in its etiology, physiology, and clinical manifestations when compared to older children and adults. Structural heart disease is the most common cause of heart failure in the newborn period, causing either pulmonary overcirculation, low cardiac output syndrome or both. Most anatomic defects that cause heart failure, fortunately, can be surgically palliated if not repaired. Functionally, the neonatal myocardium generates less contractile force and exhibits less compliance than the more mature myocardium. Despite this difference, cardiac output in the neonate may be augmented with increased filling, higher heart rate, and inotropic stimulation. Treating heart failure in this population can be quite challenging for the clinician. In general, evidence for the treatment of decompensated heart failure in the newborn is lacking. Further study in the field of pediatric heart failure, including neonates, is necessary.

References

1. Rudolph AM, Drorbaugh JE, Auld PA et al (1961) Studies on the circulation in the neonatal period. The circulation in the respiratory distress syndrome. Pediatrics 27:551-566.

2. Clyman RI, Mauray F, Wong L et al (1978) The developmental response of the ductus arteriosus to oxygen. Biol Neonate 34:177-181.
3. Oberhansli-Weis I, Heymann MA, Rudolph AM, Melmon KL (1972) The pattern and mechanism of response to oxygen by the ductus arteriosus and umbilical artery. Ped Res 6:693-700.
4. Clyman RI, Waleh N, Black SM et al (1998) Regulations of ductus arteriosus patency by nitric oxide in fetal lambs: the role of gestation, oxygen tension, and vasa vasorum. Ped Res 43:633-644.
5. Friedman WF, Printz MP, Kirkpatrick SE, Hoskins EJ (1983) The vasoactivity of the fetal lamb ductus arteriosus studied in utero. Ped Res 17:331-337.
6. Meyer WW, Lind J (1966) The ductus venosus and the mechanism of its closure. Arch Dis Child41:597-605.
7. Adeagbo AS, Coceani F, Olley PM (1982) The response of the lamb ductus venosus to prostaglandins and inhibitors of prostaglandin and thromboxane. Circ Res 51:580-586.
8. Heyman MA, Rudolph AM. Effects of congenital heart disease on fetal and neonatal circulations. Prog Cardiovasc Dis. 1972;15:115–143.
9. Cook CD, Drinker PA, Jacobson HN et al (1963) Control of pulmonary blood flow in the foetal and newly born lamab. J Physiol 169:10-29.
10. Teitel DF, Iwamoto HS, Rudolph AM (1990) Changes in the pulmonary circulation during birth-related events. Ped Res 27:372-378.
11. Anversa P, Olivetti G, Loud AV (1980) Morphometric study of early postnatal development in the left and right ventricular myocardium of the rat. Circ Res 46:495-502.
12. Korecky B, Rakusan K (1978) Normal and hypertrophic growth of the rat heart: changes in cell dimension and number. Am J Physiol 234:H123.
13. Englemann GL, Dionne CA, Jaye MC (1993) Acidic fibroblast growth factor and heart development. Role in myocyte proliferation and capillary angiogenesis. Circ Res 72:7-19.
14. Zak R (1974) Development and proliferative capacity of cardiac muscle cells. Circ Res 35(SuppII):17-2 6.
15. Weiner HL and Swain JL (1989) Acidic fibroblast growth factor mRNA is expressed by cardiac myocytes in culture and the protein is localized to the extracellular matrix. Proc Natl AcadU SA86:26 83-2687.
16. Simpson P (1985) Stimulation of hypertrophy of cultured neonatal rat heart cells through an alpha 1-adrenergic receptor and induction of beating through an alpha 1- and beta 1-adrenergic receptor interaction. Evidence for independent regulation of growth and beating. Circ Res 56:884-894.
17. Nassar R, Reedy MC, Anderson PAW (1987) Developmental changes in the ultrastructure and sarcomere shortening of the isolated rabbit ventricular myocyte. Circ Res 61:465-483.
18. Sheridan DJ, Cullen MJ, Tynan MJ (1979) Qualitative and quantitative observations on ultrastructural changes during postnatal development in the cat myocardium. J Mol Cell Cardiol 11:1173-1181.
19. Hoerter J, Mazet F, Vassort G (1981) Perinatal growth of the rabbit cardiac cell. Possible implications for the mechanism of relaxation. J Mol Cell Cardiol 13:725-740.
20. Olivetti G, Anversa P, Loud AV (1980) Morphometric study of early postnatal development in the left and right ventricular myocardium of the rat. Tissue composition, capillary growth, and sarcoplasmic alterations. Circ Res 46:503-512.
21. Fisher DJ, Heymann MA, Rudolph AM (1980) Myocardial oxygen and carbohydrate consumption in fetal lambs in utero and in adult sheep. Am J Phys 238:H399-H405.
22. Warshaw JB, Terry ML (1970) Cellular energy metabolism during fetal development. II. Fatty acid oxidation by the developing heart. J Cell Biol 44:354-360.
23. Wittels B, Bressler R (1965) Lipid metabolism in the newborn heart. J Clin Invest 44:1639-1646.

24. Swynghedauw B (1986) Developmental and functional adaptation of contractile proteins in cardiac and skeletal muscles. Physiol Rev 66:710-771.
25. Hatem SN, Sweeten T, Vetter V, Morad M (1995) Evidence for presence of Ca^{2+} stores in neonatal human atrial myocytes. Am J Physiol 268:H1195-H1201.
26. Roca TP, Pigott JD, Clarkson CW, Crumb WJ (1996) L-type calcium current in pediatric and adult human atrial myocytes: evidence for developmental changes in channel inactivation. Pediatr Res 40:462-468.
27. Mahony L, Jones LR (1986) Developmental changes in cardiac sarcoplasmic reticulum in sheep. J Biol Chem 261:15257-65.
28. Anderson RH, Baker EJ, Macartney FJ et al (2002) Myocardium and development in paediatric cardiology. Harcourt Publishers, London, 2nd edition.
29. Kitten GT, Markwald RR, Bolender DL (1987) Distribution of basement membrane antigens in cryopreserved early embryonic hearts. Anatomical Record 217:379-390.
30. Little CD, Piquet DM, Davis LA et al (1989) Distribution of laminin, collagen type IV, collagen type I, and fibronectin in chicken cardiac jelly basement membrane. Anatomical Record 224:417-425.
31. Price RL, Nakagawa M, Terracio L, Borg TK (1992) Ultrastructural localization of laminin onin vivo embryonic neonatal and adult rate cardiac myocytes and in early rat embryos raised in whole embryo culture. J Histochem and Cytochem 40:1373-1381.
32. Legato MJ (1979) Cellular mechanisms of normal growth in the mammalian heart. Qualitative and quantitative features of ventricular architecture in the dog from birth to five months of age. Circ Res 44:250-262.
33. Davies P, Dewar J, Tynan M (1975) Post-natal developmental changes in the length-tension relationship of cat papillary muscles. J Physiol 253:95-102.
34. Friedman WF, Lesch M, Sonnenblick EH (1973) Neonatal heart disease. New York: Grune and Stratton, 1973, p. 21-49.
35. Hoerter J (1976) Changes in the sensitivity to hypoxia and glucose deprivation in the isolated perfused rabbit heart during perinatal development. Pfluegers Arch 363:1-6.
36. Hopkins SF, Jr., McCutcheon EP, Wekstein DR (1973) Postnatal changes in rat ventricular function. Circ Res 32:685-691.
37. Park MK, Sheridan PH, Morgan WW, Beck N (1980) Comparative inotropic response of newborn and adult rabbit papillary muscles to isoproterenol and calcium. Dev Pharmacol Ther 1:70-82.
38. Friedman WF (1972) The intrinsic physiologic properties of the developing heart. Prog Cardiovasc Dis 15:87-111.
39. Anderson PA, Manring A, Glick KL, Crenshaw CC (1982) Biophysics of the developing heart. A comparison of the left ventricular dynamics of the fetal and neonatal lamb heart. Am J Obstet Gynecol 143:195-203.
40. Teitel DF, Sidi DD, Chin T et al (1985) Developmental changes in myocardial contractile reserve in the lamb. Pediatr Res 19:948-955.
41. Eliot RJ, Lam R, Leake RD et al (1980) Plasma catecholamine concentrations in infants at birth and during the first 48 hours of life. J Pediatr 96:311-315.
42. Gilbert RD (1982) Effects of afterload and baroreceptors on cardiac function in fetal sheep. J Dev Physiol 4:299-309.
43. Mahony L (1996) Calcium homeostasis and control of contractility in the developing heart. Semin Perinatol 20:510-519.
44. Spotnitz WD, Spotnitz HM, Truccone NJ (et al) (1979) Relation of ultrastructure and function. Sarcomere dimensions, pressure-volume curves, and geometry of the intact left ventricle of the immature canine heart. Circ Res 44:679-691.
45. Romero T, Covell J, Friedman WF (1972) A comparison of pressure-volume relations of the fetal, newborn, and adult heart. Am J Phys 222:1285-1290.

46. Nakazawa M, Miyagawa S, Ohno T et al (1988) Developmental hemodynamic changes in rat embryos at 11 to 15 days of gestation: normal data of blood pressure and the effect of caffeine compared to data from chick embryo. Pedtr Res 23:200-205.
47. Reed KL, Sahn DJ, Scagnelli S et al (1986) Doppler echocardiographic studies of diastolic function in the human fetal heart: changes during gestation. J Am Coll Cardiol 8:391-395.
48. Wladimiroff JW, Huisman TW, Stewart PA et al (1992) Normal fetal Doppler inferior vena cava, transtricuspid and umbilical artery flow velocity waveforms between 11 and 16 weeks' gestation. Am J Obstet Gynecol 166:921-924.
49. Hu N, Connuck DM, Keller BB, Clark EB (1991) Diastolic filling characteristics in the stage 12 to 27 chick embryo ventricle. Pediatr Res 29:334-7
50. Kirkpatrick SE, Pitlick PT, Naliboff J, Friedman WF (1976) Frank-Starling relationship as an important determinant of fetal cardiac output. Am J Physiol 231:495-500.
51. Romero TE, Friedman WF (1979) Limited left ventricular response to volume overload in the neonatal period: a comparative study with the adult animal. Pediatr Res13:910-5
52. Anderson PA, Killam AP, Mainwaring RD, Oakeley AE (1987) In utero right ventricular output in the fetal lamb: the efect of heart rate. J Physiol 387:297-316.
53. Anderson PA, Glick KL, Killam AP, Mainwaring RD (1986) The effect of heart rate on in utero left ventricular output in the fetal sheep. J Physiol 372:557-573.
54. Geis WP, Tatooles CJ, Priola DV, Friedman WF (1975) Factors influencing neurohormonal control of the heart in the newborn dog. Am J Physiol 228:1685-1689.
55. Friedman WF, Pool PE, Jacobowitz D et al (1968) Sympathetic innervation of the developing rabbit heart: Biochemical and histochemical comparisons of fetal, neonatal, and adult myocardium. Circ Res 23:25-32.
56. Lebowitz EA, Novich JS, Rudolph AM (1972) Development of myocardial sympathetic innervations in the fetal lamb. Pediatr Res 6:887-893.
57. Erath HG Jr, Boerth RC, Graham TP Jr (1982) Functional significance of reduced cardiac sympathetic innervation in the newborn dog. Am J Physiol 243:H20-6.
58. Booker PD (2002). Pharmacological support for childrenn with myocardial dysfunction. Paediatric Anesthesia 12:5-25.
59. Allen E, Pettigrew A, Frank D et al (1997) Alterations in dopamine clearance and catechol-O-methyltransferase activity by dopamine infusions in children. Crit Care Med 25:181-189.
60. Nottemran DA, Greenwald BM, Moran F et al (1990) Dopamine clearance in critically ill infants and children: effect of age and organ system dysfuntion. Clin Pharmacol Ther 48:138-147.
61. Lawless S, Burckart G, Diven W et al (1989) Amrinone in neonates and infants after cardiac surgery. Crit Care Med 17:751-754.
62. Ramamoorthy C, Anderson GD, Williams GD et al (1998) Pharmacokinetics and side effects of milrinone in infants and children after open heart surgery. Anesth Analg 86:283-289.
63. Wettrell G (1977) Distribution and elimination of digoxin in infants. Eur J Clin Pharmacol 11:329-335.
64. Schwartz PH, Eldadah MK, Newth CJ (1991) The pharmacokinetics of dobutamine in pediatric intensive care. Drug Metab Dispos 19:614-619.
65. Kuznetsov V, Pak E, Robinson RB et al (1995) β_2-adrenergic receptor actions in neonatal and adult rat ventricular myocytes. Cir Res 76:40-52.
66. Bartel S, Karczewski P, Krause EG (1996) G proteins, adenylyl cyclase and related phosphoproteins in the developing rat heart. Mol Cell Biochem 163/164:31-38.
67. Giannuzzi CE, Seidler FJ, Slotkin TA (1995) Beta-adrenoceptor control of cardiac adenylyl cyclase during development: agonist pre-treatment in the neonate uniquely causes heterologous sensitization, not desensitization. Brain Res 694:271-278.
68. Zeiders JL, Seidler FJ, Iaccarino G et al (1999) Ontogeny of cardiac beta-adrenoceptor desensitization mechanisms: agonist treatment enhances receptor/G-protein transduction rather than eliciting ncoupling J Mol Cell Cardiol 31:413-423.

69. Zeiders JL, Seidler FJ, Slotkin TA (1999) Agonist-induced sensitization of β-adrenoceptor signaling in neonatal rat heart:expression and catalytic activity of adenylyl cyclase. J Pharmacol Exp Ther 291:503-510.
70. Auman JT, Seidler FJ, Slotkin TA (2002) β-adrenoceptor control of G protein function in the neonate: Determinant of desensitization or sensitization. Am J Physiol Regul Integr Comp Physiol283:1236-1244.
71. Ross RD, Daniels SR, Schwartz DC et al (1987) Plasma norepinephrine levels in infants and children with congestive heart failure. Am J Cardiol 59:911-4.
72. Wu JR, Chang HR, Huang TY et al (1996) Reduction in lymphocyte beta-adrenegic receptor density in infants and children with heart failure secondary to congenital heart disease. Am J Cardiol77:170-4.
73. Price JF, Towbin JA, Denfield SW et al (2004) Arginine vasopressin levels are elevated and correlate with functional status in infants and children with congestive heart failure. Circulation 109:2550-3.
74. Kikuchi K, Nishioka K, Ueda T et al (1987) Relationship between plasma atrial natriuretic polypeptide concentration and hemodynamic measurements in children with congenital heart disease. J Pediatr 111:335-42.
75. Kunii Y, Kamada M, Ohtsuki S et al (2003) Plasma brain natriuretic peptide and the evaluation of volume overload in infants and children with congenital heart disease. Acta Med Okayama 57:191-197.
76. Jobes DR, Nicholson SC, Steven JM, Miller M, Jacobs ML, Norwood WI Jr (1992). Carbon dioxide prevents pulmonary overcirculation in hypoplastic left heart syndrome. Ann Thorac Surg54:150-151.
77. Tabbutt S, Ramamoorthy C, Montenegro LM, Durning SM, Kurth CD, Steven JM, Godinez RI, Spray TL, Wernovsky G, Nicholson SC (2001). Impact of inspired gas mixtures on preoperative infants with hypoplastic left heart syndrome during controlled ventilation. Circulation 104;I159-I164.
78. Acosta B, DiBenedetto R, Rahimi A et al.(2000) Hemodynamic effects of noninvasive bilevel positive airway pressure on patients with chronic congestive heart failure with systolic dysfunction. Chest 118:1004-1009.
79. McCrindle BW, Blackstone EH, Williams WG et al (2001) Are outcomes of surgical versus transcatheter balloon valvotomy equivalent in neonatal critical aortic stenosis? Circulation 104(12Suppl1):I152- 8.
80. Morse PM, Rockenmacher S, Pyeritz RE, Sanders SP, Bieber FR, Lin A, MacLeod P, Hall B, Graham, Jr, JM (1990) Diagnosis and management of infantile Marfan syndrome. Pediatrics 86:888-895.
81. Case RB, Morrow AG, Stainsby W, Nestor JO (1958). Anomalous origin of the left coronary artery: The physiologic defect and suggested surgical treatment. Circulation 17:1062-1068.
82. Wesselhoeft H, Fawcett JS, Johnson AL (1968). Anomalous origin of the left coronary artery from the pulmonary trunk: Its clinical spectrum, pathology, and pathophysiology, based on a review of 140 cases with seven further cases. Circulation 38:403-425.
83. Arciniegas E, Farooki ZQ, Hakimi M, Green EW (1980) Management of anomalous left coronary artery from the pulmonary artery. Circulation 62:I180-I189.
84. Kakou GM, Sidi D, Kachaner J, Villain E, Cohen L, Piechaud JF, Le Bidois J, Pedroni E, Vouhe P, Neveux JY (1988) Anomalous left coronary artery arising from the pulmonary artery in infancy: is early operation better? Br Heart J 60:522-526.
85. Carvalho JS, Redington AN, Oldershaw PJ, Shinebourne EA, Lincoln CR, Gibson DG (1991). Analysis of left ventricular wall movement before and after reimplantation of anomalous left coronary artery in infancy. Br Heart J 65:218-222.
86. Adams KF, Fonarow GC, Emerman CL et al (2005) In-hospital mortality in patients with acute decompensated heart failure requiring intravenous vasoactive medications: an analysis

from the Acute Decompensated Heart Failure National Registry (ADHERE). J Am Coll Cardiol46:57-64 .
87. Cuffe MS, Califf RM, Adams KF et al (2002). Short-term intravenous milrinone for acute exacerbation of chronic heart failure: a randomized controlled trial. JAMA 287: 1541-1547.
88. Felker MG, Benza RL, Chandler AB et al (2003) Heart failure etiology and response to milrinone in decompensated heart failure: results from the OPTIME-CHF study. J Am Coll Cardiol 41:997-1003.
89. Chang AC, Atz AM, Wernovsky G et al (1995) Milrinone: Systemic and pulmonary emodynamic effects in neonates after cardiac surgery. Crit Care Med 23:1907-1914.
90. Teshima H, Tobita K, Yamamura H et al (2002) Cardiovascular effects of a phosphodiesterase III inhibitor, amrinone, in infants: Non-invasive echocardiographic evaluation. Pediatr Int 44:259-263.
91. Hoffman TM, Wernovsky G, Atz AM et al (2003) Efficacy and safety of milrinone in preventing low cardiac output syndrome in infants and children after corrective surgery for congenital heart disease. Circulation 107:996-1002.
92. Leier CV, Webel J, Bush CA (1977) The cardiovascular effects of the continuous infusion of dobutamine in patients with severe cardiac failure. Circulation 56:468-472.
93. O'Connor CM, Gattis WA, Uretsky BF et al (1999) Continuous intravenous dobutamine is associated with an increased risk of death in patients with advanced heart failure: insights from the Flolan International Randomized Survival Trial (FIRST). Am Heart J 138:78-86.

Chronic Heart Failure in Children with Congenital Heart Disease

3

Kimberly Y. Lin and Robert E. Shaddy

Surgical therapy for children born with congenital heart disease has improved survival enormously in this group of patients. Children who were once expected to die either before or immediately after surgery, now enjoy longevity that 20 years ago was unheard of.[1] Now that perioperative mortality has been reduced to very low levels in most complex cardiac lesions, this group of patients has entered into pediatric cardiology clinical care with a relatively new set of needs. These needs include the monitoring and treatment of rhythm abnormalities, valve abnormalities, and ventricular myocardial abnormalities. Derangement in any of these closely linked systems can cause, or at least be associated with, the development of chronic heart failure. Although the recognition and definition of heart failure in this patient population may not be precisely defined as of yet, it is clear that many of these patients will develop signs and symptoms of heart failure. It is incumbent on those of us caring for these patients that we work diligently to develop an evidence base from which to treat these patients. Although a large evidence base exists for the treatment of chronic heart failure in the adult, similar evidence-based guidelines in children are lacking.[2,3]

Large multicenter trials have defined a therapeutic approach to the adult with chronic heart failure. These trials have resulted in recommendations from the American Heart Association (AHA), the American College of Cardiology (ACC), and the Heart Failure Society of America (HFSA).[2] Tables 3.1 and 3.2 provide a summary of the recommendations put forth by the AHA and ACC for adult patients with current or prior symptoms of heart failure. Class I recommendations reflect conditions for which there is evidence and/or general agreement that a given procedure or treatment is beneficial, useful, and effective. Class II recommendations reflect conditions for which there is conflict regarding the usefulness or efficacy of a procedure or treatment; these are further subdivided into Class IIa (weight of evidence or opinion is in favor of usefulness or efficacy) and Class IIb (usefulness or efficacy is less well established by evidence or opinion). Finally, Class III recommendations reflect conditions for which there is evidence and/or general agreement that a procedure or treatment is not useful or effective, and in some cases may be harmful. The level of evidence supporting each recommendation is listed as either A (data derived from multiple randomized clinical trials or meta-analyses), B (data derived from a single

K.Y. Lin (✉)
The Children's Hospital of Philadelphia, University of Pennsylvania School of Medicine, Philadelphia, PA

R.E. Shaddy (ed.), *Heart Failure in Congenital Heart Disease*,
DOI: 10.1007/978-1-84996-480-7_3, © Springer-Verlag London Limited 2011

Table 3.1 Medical treatment recommendations for adults with current or prior symptoms of heart failure (Stage C)

Class I	Class IIa	Class IIb	Class III
Diuretics if fluid retention (LOE:C)	*ARBs* as alternative to ACEIs, especially if already on ARBs (LOE:A)	Addition of *ARBs* can be considered in patients with persistent symptoms on optimal therapy (LOE:B)	Routine combined use of *ACEI*, *ARB* and *aldosterone antagonist* (LOE:C)
ACEI unless contraindicated (LOE:A)	*Digitalis* for treatment of symptoms unless contraindicated (LOE:B)	*Hydralazine and a nitrate* in patients who cannot take ACEI or ARB (LOE:C)	*Calcium channel blockers* (LOE:A)
ARBs if ACEI-intolerant (LOE:A)	*Hydralazine and a nitrate* in patients already on ACEI and beta-blocker with persistent symptoms (LOE:A)		Long-term intermittent infusion of *positive inotropic drugs* (LOE:C)
Beta-blockers unless contraindicated (LOE:A)			Routine use of *nutritional supplements* or *hormones* (LOE:C)
Aldosterone antagonists in patients with NYHA III-IV, preserved renal function, and normal serum potassium (LOE:B)			
Exercise training in ambulatory patients (LOE:B)			

Adapted from [2] with permission. *LOE* level of evidence, *ACEI* angiotensin converting enzyme inhibitor, *ARB* angiotensin II receptor blocker, *NYHA* New York Heart Association (Class I-IV), *LVEF* left ventricular ejection fraction

Table 3.2 Device recommendations for adults with current or prior symptoms of heart failure (StageC)

ClassI	ClassI Ia
ICDs Secondary prevention in patients with reduced LVEF and history of cardiac arrest, ventricular fibrillation or destabilizing ventricular tachycardia (LOE:A) Primary prevention in ischemic heart disease with LVEF ≤ 30%, NYHA II-III, on optimal medical therapy (LOE:A) Primary prevention in nonischemic cardiomyopathy with LVEF ≤ 30%, NYHA II-III, on optimal medical therapy (LOE:B)	*ICDs* in patients with LVEF 30–35% of any origin, NYHA II-III, on optimal medical therapy (LOE:B)
CRT in patients with LVEF ≤ 35%, NYHA III-IV, and QRS >120 ms on optimal medical therapy (LOE:A)	

Adapted from [2] with permission. *ICD* implantable cardioverter-defibrillator, *LOE* level of evidence, *LVEF* left ventricular ejection fraction, *NYHA* New York Heart Association (Class I-IV), *CRT* cardiac resynchronization therapy

randomized trial, or nonrandomized studies, or C (only consensus opinion of experts, case studies, or standard-of-care).

The ACC/AHA recommendations for adults with heart failure shown in Tables 3.1 and 3.2 include medications such as diuretics (for fluid overload), angiotensin converting enzyme (ACE) inhibitors, angiotensin receptor blockers (ARBs), beta-adrenergic receptor (beta) blockers, aldosterone antagonists, and digoxin. Device therapies, including cardiac resynchronization therapy (CRT), and implantable cardioverter-defibrillators (ICDs) have also been shown to be efficacious in the management of chronic congestive heart failure in adults. The efficacy of these pharmacologic and device therapies are based on large, prospective, randomized trials in adults. It is safe to assume that few if any of the tens of thousands of patients enrolled in these adult heart failure trials had a diagnosis of structural congenital heart disease. Indeed, most of these patients had ischemic heart disease, and the remainder had dilated cardiomyopathy.

This chapter will review what is known about chronic heart failure in patients with congenital heart disease and will provide a framework for thinking of these patients as a group of patients either at risk for heart failure, having pre-symptomatic cardiac abnormalities, having overt chronic heart failure, and ultimately having end-stage heart failure. The authors will provide recommendations for monitoring and treatment of such individuals. Since other chapters in this book will focus on heart failure in patients with a systemic right ventricle, and on device therapy in congenital heart disease, discussions of these topics will be limited.

3.1 Heart Failure Due to Left-to-Right Shunt Lesions

Patients with large left-to-right intracardiac shunts have pulmonary overcirculation, and have traditionally been described as being in heart failure. These lesions include left-to-right intracardiac shunts at all cardiac levels: unobstructed anomalous pulmonary venous connection, atrial level shunt, atrioventricular level shunt, ventricular level shunt, proximal aortopulmonary connections, and patent ductus arteriosus. At one time, newborn repair of all but the most simple lesions (e.g., patent ductus arteriosus) was a high risk procedure and attempts to medically manage these patients was commonplace. However, most major medical centers in developed countries now routinely surgically correct these lesions as needed early in childhood, and thus require minimal medical management.

Medical treatment strategies have traditionally included diuretics and digoxin, with more recent studies suggesting benefit from ACE inhibitors and beta-blockers. Diuretics are a common medication used to treat symptomatic patient with large left-to-right shunts. Although there are no studies supporting or refuting their use, it intuitively makes sense, and the immediate benefits of diuretics can be seen in children with this physiology. Diuretics reduce ventricular filling pressures, atrial pressures, and lung water. Digoxin has been used in this group of patient with mixed results. Some studies have shown potential benefit, others no effect, and still others have shown possible deleterious effects acutely in the setting of left-to-right intracardiac shunts.[4–7] Soon after ACE inhibitors were starting to be used in children for hypertension, several studies in animals and in humans with ventricular level shunts suggested possible benefit from ACE inhibitors, presumably due to their relatively selective effect of afterload reduction on the systemic circulation, thus increasing systemic blood flow and reducing pulmonary blood flow.[8–12] There is no good data available on the utility of ARBs on this group of patients. After the approval of beta-blockers for the treatment of heart failure in adults, a group in Germany began exploring the utility of these drugs on children with large left-to right shunts and failure to thrive. In a series of studies, they were able to demonstrate significant benefit from beta-blockers in this group of patients from the standpoint of improved neurohormonal profiles, decreased respiratory symptoms and improved growth.[13–17] Although these pharmacologic interventions may not be necessary in institutions where early surgical intervention can be performed with low risk and high success, there may be co-morbidities (e.g., extreme prematurity) that may warrant initiation of such therapies. In addition, in developing countries where surgical options are limited, there may be a strong role for the use of these medications, particularly in infants with moderate-size ventricular septal defects that often get smaller over time if the infant is able to thrive.

3.2 Systemic Left Ventricular Dysfunction

Systemic left ventricle (LV) dysfunction can occur either in association with unoperated congenital heart disease, or after repair of congenital heart disease (CHD). In unoperated congenital heart disease, it is not uncommon for the LV to demonstrate either dilatation, systolic dysfunction, diastolic dysfunction, or some combination of all three of these entities. The diagnosis is usually easily made by echocardiography, and this information may be critical to deciding type and timing of surgical or transcatheter treatment of the congenital heart lesion. For instance, in patients with aortic or mitral valve disease, the assessment and at times, the treatment of LV dilatation or dysfunction may be crucial for deciding preoperative management and timing of surgery. Other more common lesions such as ventricular septal defect or patent ductus arteriosus may have the typical LV dilation associated with these left-to-right shunt lesions, but occasionally also have LV dysfunction that may be unexplained. An increased diagnosis of LV noncompaction has also been seen in patients with congenital heart disease.[18] Of course, sometimes the associated congenital heart lesion may be an unimportant bystander to a cardiomyopathy, such as a small VSD in a patient with idiopathic dilated cardiomyopathy. Much of the surveillance clinical visits, including echocardiography, that is done in patients with unoperated CHD is directed toward monitoring LV performance, and may ultimately dictate initiation of medical and/or surgical treatment.

Systemic LV dysfunction after surgical palliation or repair of a congenital heart defect is much less common in the current era. The reasons for this are multifactorial, including improved methods of cardiac preservation during cardiopulmonary bypass, shorter surgical duration, and less need for ventriculotomies. Hypothermia and cardioplegia are the mainstays of myocardial protection for children during bypass surgery, although the optimal timing, degree, and specific components of these strategies remain a topic of much debate.[19,20] When ventriculotomy is required, an apical approach when feasible may preserve LV function better than a longitudinal incision.[21]

In the first 24–36 h after cardiac surgery, patients often experience a period of low cardiac output that requires multiple supportive measures in the intensive care unit. The PRIMACORP study randomized post-operative pediatric patients to placebo or one of two doses of milrinone.[22] In this landmark study, milrinone decreased the incidence of postoperative low cardiac output syndrome and has now been adopted by many cardiac intensive care units as standard treatment for children after repair of CHD. If ischemia is thought to be a contributing cause to postoperative LV dysfunction, management is primarily based upon individual circumstance and adult data (see section on ischemic cardiomyopathy). Diagnostic studies such as aortic and coronary angiography may be necessary to confirm or exclude ischemic compromise after CHD surgery in a child with post-operative LV dysfunction. Beyond the immediate postoperative period, management of chronic LV dysfunction in children should follow similar treatment protocols to adults with chronic heart failure, including diuretics for fluid overload, ACE inhibitors, beta-blockers, aldosterone antagonists, and digoxin for symptomatic heart failure.[23,24] Cardiac resynchronization therapy and implantable cardioverter-defibrillators should also be considered part of our armamentarium for the treatment of these children, although the indications for their use is much less clear than in adults.[25–28]

Growing interest is being given to the morphologic LV in l-transposition of the great arteries (l-TGA, also referred to as congenitally corrected transposition). The combined atrial and arterial switch operation can now relieve the morphologic right ventricle of the work of pumping blood to the systemic circulation, placing the morphologic left ventricle in its place.[29] Unless substantial pulmonary hypertension or an unrestrictive VSD are present, the morphologic LV must be "trained" with a pulmonary artery band before undergoing the full double switch operation. Much debate remains, however, regarding whether the morphologic LV can be artificially prepared for systemic use in this circumstance. Early results were promising, but longer term studies now show a significant number of double switch patients with LV dysfunction.[30,31] In the current era, this operation is usually performed at centers that can support cardiac transplantation in cases where the LV fails. Even for those patients who initially do well, long-term monitoring of ventricular function is necessary. Older age at the time of preparatory pulmonary arterial banding appears to be one risk factor for LV dysfunction after the double switch procedure.[32] Some believe that this is because an older heart responds to outflow tract obstruction with more hypertrophy than hyperplasia, analogous to systemic hypertension and LV hypertrophy. Others suspect that LV failure will decrease as the surgical techniques improve. Improved surgical technique may lead to less neo-aortic insufficiency that can be caused by the pulmonary artery band. Surgical innovations such as an adjustable pulmonary artery band may allow a more gradual pressure load to be placed on the morphologic LV. The double switch procedure holds great promise, but more long term studies are needed before it can be universally recommended to all patients with congenitally corrected transposition of the great arteries.

There is little data to guide management of children with hemodynamically-compromising and/or acutely decompensated LV dysfunction. Supportive care with inotropic support should be instituted when there is chance of recovering adequate LV function, or when cardiac transplantation is an option. Multiple modes of mechanical circulatory support have been used successfully in children, including extracorporeal membrane oxygenator (ECMO) circuits, intra-aortic balloon pumps (IABP), and various ventricular assist devices (VAD).[33] Please see the chapters on mechanical circulatory support and indications and outcomes of heart transplantation for further information on these therapies in children.

3.3 Ischemic Cardiomyopathies

Ischemic cardiomyopathy is much less common in children with heart failure than in adults. However, there are several congenital abnormalities and common complications of interventions upon them which can lead to ischemic heart disease. These conditions include anomalous left coronary artery from the pulmonary artery (ALCAPA), anomalous aortic origin of a coronary artery (AAOCA), pulmonary autograft replacement for the aortic valve (Ross procedure), and the arterial switch operation (ASO) for transposition of the great arteries. The abnormal origin or manipulation of the coronary arteries at their origins puts them at risk of ostial stenosis as well as arterial kinking, stretching, and narrowing.[34] Careful preoperative assessment that delineates the origins and courses of the coronary arteries is vital to planning a surgical intervention that involves reimplantation of the coronary arteries. In fact, some series have shown that any variation in coronary anatomy is a predictor of outcome in ASO surgery, while others show higher rates of ischemia with only the intramural coronary variants.[35–37]

Anomalous origin of the coronary arteries is a congenital heart defect that usually requires surgical intervention. Infants with ALCAPA develop symptoms when their pulmonary vascular resistance drops, and therefore, coronary artery perfusion is compromised. These children are often quite ill with severely depressed LV function, and require urgent surgical correction. Recovery of LV myocardial function appears to be quite good in the modern era after dual coronary artery surgical repair for ALCAPA. Schwartz et al reported normalization of LV function in all 28 ALCAPA patients who had follow-up beyond 1 year after surgery in their series.[38] Preoperative LV function did not predict outcome, lending credence to the idea that hibernating myocardium exists in patients with chronic ischemia. This leaves open the possibility of full myocardial recovery after revascularization.[39,40] The degree of preoperative mitral regurgitation, however, has been described as a risk factor for mortality.[38] While LV dysfunction with associated chamber enlargement is usually the underlying mechanism for mitral regurgitation in ALCAPA, consideration for intervention on the mitral valve should be given in cases of severe preoperative mitral regurgitation. Postoperatively, LV function may take weeks to months to recover. Left ventricular assist devices have been used in the immediate postoperative period for those patients who cannot be separated from cardiopulmonary bypass.[41,42]

In congenital heart surgical procedures which require reimplantation of the coronary arteries, postoperative heart failure symptoms and ventricular dysfunction have long been attributed to anatomical problems with coronary blood flow. While this is certainly a major contributing factor in most cases of ischemic cardiomyopathy after coronary reimplantation, some studies suggest that sympathetic denervation may also play a role.[43,44] Kondo et al. showed that sympathetic reinnervation occurred in all patients who had an ASO in early infancy, but was variable in patients who went for ASO at an older age. They also showed a negative relationship between cardiac denervation and exercise performance, lending clinical relevance to their findings. This should be taken into consideration when the timing of a child's coronary reimplantation surgery is in question. Others have shown that denervation of the proximal coronary arteries after ASO may cause long-term abnormalities in coronary artery growth, vascular reserve and function.[45] While there is no data on denervation and coronary development after the Ross procedure, this ASO data suggests that long-term follow up of children after any coronary reimplantation surgery is important.

The diagnosis of ischemic cardiomyopathy in children, as in adults, lies primarily with ECG, echocardiography, and clinical history. Blood tests to look for markers of myocardial ischemia such as troponin I, troponin T, and creatine kinase (CK)-MB may be helpful, although the trend may be more useful than the absolute value in postoperative cases where some myocardial injury is expected at baseline. Other possible diagnostic tests include stress tests, computerized tomography (CT), magnetic resonance imaging (MRI), and nuclear perfusion scans. Although stress tests may provide some useful diagnostic information, they should be interpreted with caution, as a negative stress test does not necessarily exclude the possibility of anomalous coronary arteries.[46] Daniels suggests the following criteria for using stress tests: (1) High index of suspicion after initial work up; (2) Structurally normal heart; (3) Patient able to cooperate with medical or exercise-induced stress testing.[47] Nuclear perfusion imaging may be useful for delineating perfusion defects and regional wall motion abnormalities. In their series of patients undergoing repair for anomalous aortic origin of a coronary artery (AAOCA), Brothers et al found that it took a combination of three modalities – exercise stress test, stress echocardiogram, and myocardial perfusion scan – to identify ischemia in patients who were often asymptomatic.[48] CT and MRI may also be of benefit for delineating coronary anatomy. When the aforementioned modalities do not clearly point to a diagnosis of ischemia despite high clinical suspicion, cardiac catheterization with selective coronary angiography remains the gold standard.

The management of children with these and other conditions affecting coronary blood flow to the myocardium is almost completely extrapolated from adult data. The guidelines for management of adults after myocardial infarction include a host of medications with Class I indications, including beta-blockers, ACE inhibitors, HMG-CoA reductase inhibitors (statins), nitroglycerin for anginal symptoms, aspirin, and clopidogrel.[49,50] Most of these medications have not been studied in children and adults with congenital heart disease and ischemic cardiomyopathy, so their application in this circumstance must be considered in context of the underlying disease process. Beta-blockers, if clinically tolerated, should be considered for their beneficial effects on heart rate as well as neurohormonal activation. ACE inhibitors should likewise be considered for their cardiac remodeling benefits if the patient's blood pressure will allow their use. Unless an atherosclerotic process is suspected, statins do not have a clear role in this patient population, although evidence of a beneficial anti-inflammatory effect even in the absence of elevated LDL cholesterol levels is growing.[51,52] While there is little data to direct what level of antiplatelet agents should be used in these patients to prevent coronary artery thrombosis, most practitioners will place these patients on aspirin unless another agent is indicated for other reasons. Once the anatomic reason for coronary flow obstruction has been addressed, long term nitroglycerin should not be necessary in this patient population.

3.4 Heart Failure due to Valve Disease

Valve abnormalities are common in congenital heart disease and can contribute to the development and progression of heart failure in this population. Valve abnormalities can manifest as either stenosis or insufficiency/regurgitation, with the most common abnormality being a combination of both. Management of valve stenosis almost invariably involves surgical or transcatheter intervention, and medical management has a very limited role. This section will focus on management of valve insufficiency. Valve insufficiency creates a volume load on the heart, which can cause it to fail. Other changes caused by valve insufficiency, such as sympathetic activation, can also contribute to heart failure.[53] The ACC and AHA published their most recent guidelines for the management of patients with valvular heart disease in 2006, with a focused update in 2008.[54] These guidelines include a section which specifically addresses congenital valvar disease in adolescents and young adults. Heart failure due to tricuspid regurgitation and pulmonary insufficiency will be addressed elsewhere in this book. Here we will assess the data on the management of heart failure in children due to chronic mitral regurgitation and aortic insufficiency, with reference to the aforementioned guidelines where applicable.

Accurate diagnosis and quantification of valvar insufficiency is critical to determining timing and types of intervention. Transthoracic echocardiography is most commonly used in children to noninvasively determine the mechanism and severity of mitral regurgitation, as well as to measure LV size and function. Occasionally, 3-dimensional echocardiography is utilized to augment this information, especially in cases of complicated atrioventricular valve anatomy. Transesophageal echocardiography, magnetic resonance imaging (MRI), and cardiac catheterization are less commonly needed in children as compared with adults with valvar regurgitation, since adequate acoustic windows are usually present. Serial echocardiography is recommended on an annual or semiannual basis to monitor LV function in asymptomatic patients with moderate to severe mitral regurgitation.[54] Exercise testing may be useful in asymptomatic patients with severe mitral regurgitation to assess exercise tolerance and changes in pulmonary artery pressure and severity of mitral regurgitation with exertion, especially if further intervention is being considered.

The ACC/AHA guidelines list two class I recommendations for mitral valve surgery in adolescent and young adults with severe mitral regurgitation: (1) those who are symptomatic (NYHA class III or IV), and (2) asymptomatic patients with LV systolic dysfunction (ejection fraction < 0.60). These guidelines also give a class IIa recommendation for mitral valve repair in "experienced surgical centers" in asymptomatic adolescents or young adults with severe mitral regurgitation and preserved LV systolic function "if the likelihood of successful repair without residual MR is greater than 90%."[54] The delicate balance in these younger patients is to operate soon enough to avoid irreversible LV systolic dysfunction, but not so soon as to commit a young patient to repeat operations with successive prosthetic mitral valve replacements and long-term anticoagulation. There is no consensus as to the point at which LV dysfunction due to mitral regurgitation becomes irreversible. At least one series in children reports normalization of LV function in most pediatric patients after mitral valve replacement.[55] For symptomatic patients with severe mitral regurgitation and severe LV dysfunction, cardiac transplantation may also be considered.

The medical management of chronic mitral regurgitation in children with heart failure is derived almost entirely from anecdotal experience. While the efficacy of ACE inhibitors has not been conclusively shown to prevent LV dysfunction in isolated mitral regurgitation in children or adults, it is clearly indicated when heart failure is present in adults.[53,54] Several small studies support ACE inhibition specifically in children with chronic mitral regurgitation. A few reports have examined the utility of ACE inhibition in children with either mitral regurgitation and/or aortic insufficiency. These showed either clinical improvement[56] or echocardiographic improvement in LV end diastolic and end systolic dimensions as well as LV mass.[57] Calabro demonstrated that in ten asymptomatic children with chronic MR, a single dose of oral enalapril resulted in improved echocardiographic parameters.[58] However, larger and longer-term studies in children are lacking. The data in adults is equivocal with respect to ACE inhibition in asymptomatic mitral regurgitation.[59,60]

When ACE inhibition is not possible or tolerated (e.g., cough or angioedema), an angiotensin receptor blocker (ARB) can be considered. To date, there are no data regarding the efficacy of ARBs in children with heart failure and valvar insufficiency, but these medications have been used safely in children with conditions such as hypertension and nephropathy.[59] Studies in adults suggest a benefit from ARBs in mitral regurgitation, presumably due to the similarities in mechanism of action that they share with ACE inhibitors.[61] Beta blockers have shown some promise in canine models of mitral regurgitation and heart failure,[62] but have not been rigorously tested in humans for this indication. Certainly any of these agents should be considered when hypertension is present as a comorbidity in pediatric patients with heart failure.

Aortic insufficiency creates both pressure and volume loads on the LV. The pressure load results from the heart's compensatory mechanisms of increased LV end diastolic volume and increased systolic wall stress, which lead to an increase in afterload and contributes to a positive feedback loop that results in LV hypertrophy.[63] The cornerstone of evaluation for children with aortic insufficiency is transthoracic echocardiography. If the acoustic windows are not adequate, a cardiac MRI or radionuclide angiography can be used to further delineate critical information, including the degree of insufficiency, aortic valve and root morphology, and LV size and function. Cardiac catheterization can supply additional hemodynamic information, albeit in a more invasive manner. One might elect to pursue cardiac catheterization when coronary artery anatomy also needs to be clearly delineated, as in the case of a patient being considered for a Ross procedure. Exercise testing is indicated when a patient's history of symptoms is equivocal, and a functional assessment is needed for determining physical activity restrictions.[54]

Class I indications for aortic valve repair or replacement in adolescents and young adults with chronic severe aortic insufficiency include the following: (1) symptoms of angina, syncope, or dyspnea on exertion; (2) LV systolic dysfunction (EF < 50%); and (3) progressive LV enlargement.[54] Those with moderate AS (peak-to-peak gradient >40 mmHg) in addition to chronic severe AI, or with ST depression or T wave inversion on resting ECG may also be considered for aortic valve surgery (Class II indications).[54] As with any valve surgery, these indications must be taken in context of the technical difficulties related to patient size in neonates and younger children.

Vasodilator therapy to improve forward stroke volume and reduce regurgitant volume has been explored in adults with aortic insufficiency with varying results.[54] Several trials using long-acting calcium channel blockers in asymptomatic adults with chronic aortic insufficiency have yielded conflicting data on its efficacy in aortic insufficiency.[64–67] The data in adults regarding use of ACE inhibitors in aortic insufficiency are similarly inconclusive.[66,68] Given this lack of convincing evidence, the indications for the use of vasodilator therapy in adults with aortic insufficiency are quite limited: (1) severe AI with symptoms and/or LV dysfunction who are poor candidates for surgery (Class I); (2) short-term use due to severe heart failure symptoms and severe LV dysfunction while awaiting surgery (Class IIa); (3) asymptomatic patients who have LV dilatation but normal systolic function (Class IIb).[54]

Despite this paucity of evidence to support the use of vasodilators in adults with aortic insufficiency, agents such as ACE inhibitors are quite commonly used in children with aortic insufficiency. While it may be reasonable to consider ACE inhibitors in the setting of LV systolic dysfunction before aortic valve surgery, it is less clear whether these agents should be used with a goal of preventing systolic dysfunction in those with normal LV systolic function. As mentioned previously, several small studies in children reported either clinical improvement[56] or echocardiographic improvement in LV dimensions[57] with the use of ACE inhibitors. An important limitation of these studies is that they did not distinguish between children with mitral regurgitation and aortic insufficiency. In their study of 23 asymptomatic children with normal LV shortening fraction and moderate to severe AI, Alehan and Ozkutlu were able to show echocardiographic improvements after 1 year of ACE inhibition.[69] Without further data to support their use in children with aortic insufficiency and the conflicting data on this topic in adults, ACE inhibitors can certainly be considered but are not universally recommended in children with AI and preserved LV systolicf unction.

3.5 Heart Failure in Systemic Single Ventricle Patients

Patients with single ventricle physiology and heart failure are increasing in number almost as quickly as our success with single ventricle surgical palliation grows. The diagnosis of heart failure in these patients may be less straightforward than in biventricular patients because the available data is often more subjective in nature. A single ventricle patient may not have a clear history of exercise intolerance because they are often restricted in physical activity at baseline, and they may not reach target heart rate due to chronotropic impairment in the exercise laboratory. Assessment of ventricular systolic function is generally qualitative by echocardiography when the typical landmarks for calculating a shortening fraction are not available, although an ejection fraction can be calculated by echocardiography or cardiac MRI when desired. Objective measures of diastolic dysfunction in congenital heart disease, such as tissue Doppler imaging at the tricuspid valve annulus, have been validated in some centers and are now being used on a more widespread basis. Cardiac catheterization remains the gold standard for diagnostic evaluation in cases where symptoms and noninvasive imaging do not clearly identify whether a single ventricle patient has hemodynamic and/or anatomic abnormalities that could result in heart failure. Evaluation for other signs of end-organ dysfunction is paramount in such situations. The "failing Fontan physiology" may manifest as cirrhosis, renal failure, protein-losing enteropathy, or plastic bronchitis, with or without systemic ventricular dysfunction or pure heart failure symptoms.

Several small studies give mixed results with respect to the use of ACE inhibitors in patients with single ventricle physiology. Thompson et al showed that perioperative ACE inhibitors decreased the severity and duration of pleural effusions after bidirectional cavopulmonary anastomosis surgery.[70] In contrast, Kouatli et al. showed no benefit on exercise performance of ACE inhibitors after the Fontan operation.[71] Likewise, Ohuchi et al saw an impairment in cardiac autonomic activity after Fontan operation that did not improve with the administration of enalapril as compared with a control group that did not receive ACE inhibitors.[72] We look for the upcoming results of the NIH-sponsored Infants with Single Ventricle (ISV) trial for the first multicenter, randomized, controlled trial of ACE inhibitors in a single ventricle population.

The Pediatric Carvedilol Study randomized children to carvedilol, a beta blocker with additional alpha blocking activity which has been shown to improve outcomes in adults with heart failure, or to placebo. This study did not find a significant improvement in heart failure symptoms with carvedilol.[71] However, there was a significant interaction between carvedilol effect and ventricular morphology, with a trend towards less beneficial effects of carvedilol in patients with a non-morphologic LV serving as their systemic ventricle, when compared to those with a systemic LV. These results serve as a reminder that data from adult trials should not be extrapolated to patients with CHD without careful consideration, and that further studies in this patient population are sorely needed.

3.6 Summary

Advances in the surgical management of congenital heart disease over the past 50 years have been breathtaking. Nearly all of these patients, however, are at risk for or manifest some degree of heart failure in their now-extended lifetimes. While the evidence base for the management of adults with heart failure has grown tremendously in the past decade, a similar evidence base specific to patients with CHD and heart failure is merely in its infancy. We are only now starting to understand the indications for various medications and interventions in CHD patients with heart failure. ACE inhibitors in asymptomatic patients with valvar insufficiency, beta-blockers in patients with single morphologic LVs, and cardiac resynchronization therapy in children are but a few of the interventions yet to be proven to improve or not improve outcomes in CHD patients. Our ability to prevent, detect, and manage heart failure in congenital heart patients is the next frontier in pediatric cardiology.

References

1. Wernovsky G. The paradigm shift toward surgical intervention for neonates with hypoplastic left heart syndrome. *Arch Pediatr Adolesc Med.*2008; 162:849–854.
2. Hunt SA, Abraham WT, Chin MH et al. ACC/AHA 2005 Guideline update for the diagnosis and management of chronic heart failure in the Adult-Summary Article A Report of the American College of Cardiology/American Heart Association Task Force on Practice Guidelines (writing committee to update the 2001 guidelines for the evaluation and management of heart failure). *J Am Coll Cardiol.*2005; 46:1116–1143.
3. Rosenthal D, Chrisant MR, Edens E et al. International society for heart and lung transplantation: practice guidelines for management of heart failure in children. *J Heart Lung Transplant.* 2004;23:1313–1333.

4. Berman W, Jr., Yabek SM, Dillon T, Niland C, Corlew S, Christensen D. Effects of digoxin in infants with congested circulatory state due to a ventricular septal defect. *N Engl J Med.* 1983;308:363–366.
5. Redington AN, Carvalho JS, Shinebourne EA. Does digoxin have a place in the treatment of the child with congenital heart disease? *Cardiovasc Drugs Ther.*1989; 3:21–24.
6. Kimball TR, Daniels SR, Meyer RA et al. Effect of digoxin on contractility and symptoms in infants with a large ventricular septal defect. *Am J Cardiol*1991; 68:1377–1382.
7. Seguchi M, Nakazawa M, Momma K. Further evidence suggesting a limited role of digitalis in infants with circulatory congestion secondary to large ventricular septal defect. *Am J Cardiol.*1999;83:1 408–1411,A 8.
8. Shaddy RE, Teitel DF, Brett C. Short-term hemodynamic effects of captopril in infants with congestive heart failure. *Am J Dis Child.*1988; 142:100–105.
9. Montigny M, Davignon A, Fouron JC, Biron P, Fournier A, Elie R. Captopril in infants for congestive heart failure secondary to a large ventricular left-to-right shunt. *Am J Cardiol.* 1989;63:631–633.
10. Lloyd TR, Mahoney LT, Knoedel D, Marvin WJ, Jr., Robillard JE, Lauer RM. Orally administered enalapril for infants with congestive heart failure: a dose-finding study. *J Pediatr.* 1989;114:650–654.
11. Rheuban KS, Carpenter MA, Ayers CA, Gutgesell HP. Acute hemodynamic effects of converting enzyme inhibition in infants with congestive heart failure. *J Pediatr.* 1990;117:668–670.
12. Momma K. ACE inhibitors in pediatric patients with heart failure. *Paediatr Drugs.* 2006;8:55–69.
13. Buchhorn R, Bartmus D, Siekmeyer W, Hulpke-Wette M, Schulz R, Bursch J. Beta-blocker therapy of severe congestive heart failure in infants with left to right shunts. *Am J Cardiol.* 1998;81:1366–138.
14. Buchhorn R, Hulpke-Wette M, Hilgers R, Bartmus D, Wessel A, Bursch J. Propranolol treatment of congestive heart failure in infants with congenital heart disease: The CHF-PRO-INFANT Trial. Congestive heart failure in infants treated with propanol. *Int J Cardiol.* 2001;79:167–173.
15. Buchhorn R, Hulpke-Wette M, Nothroff J, Paul T. Heart rate variability in infants with heart failure due to congenital heart disease: reversal of depressed heart rate variability by propranolol. *Med Sci Monit.*2002; 8:CR661–CR666.
16. Buchhorn R, Hulpke-Wette M, Ruschewski W et al. Beta-receptor downregulation in congenital heart disease: a risk factor for complications after surgical repair? *Ann Thorac Surg.* 2002;73:610–613.
17. Buchhorn R, Hulpke-Wette M, Ruschewski W et al. Effects of therapeutic beta blockade on myocardial function and cardiac remodelling in congenital cardiac disease. *Cardiol Young.* 2003;13:36–43.
18. Pignatelli RH, McMahon CJ, Dreyer WJ et al. Clinical characterization of left ventricular noncompaction in children: a relatively common form of cardiomyopathy. Circulation 2003;108:2672–2678.
19. Doenst T, Schlensak C, Beyersdorf F. Cardioplegia in pediatric cardiac surgery: do we believe in magic? *Ann Thorac Surg.*2003; 75:1668–1677.
20. Allen BS, Barth MJ, Ilbawi MN. Pediatric myocardial protection: an overview. *Semin Thorac Cardiovasc Surg.*2001; 13:56–72.
21. DiBernardo LR, Kirshbom PM, Skaryak LA et al. Acute functional consequences of left ventriculotomy. *Ann Thorac Surg.*1998; 66:159–165.
22. Hoffman TM, Wernovsky G, Atz AM et al. Efficacy and safety of milrinone in preventing low cardiac output syndrome in infants and children after corrective surgery for congenital heart disease. *Circulation.*2003; 107:996–1002.

23. Shaddy RE, Tani LY. Chronic congestive heart failure. In: Allen HD, Driscoll DJ, Shaddy RE, Feltes T, eds. *Moss and Adams' Heart Disease in Infants, Children, and Adolescents, Including the Fetus and Young Adult.* 7th ed. Philadelphia, PA: Lippincott, Williams & Wilkins; 2007:1495–1504.
24. Hunt SA, Baker DW, Chin MH et al. ACC/AHA guidelines for the evaluation and management of chronic heart failure in the adult: executive summary a report of the American college of cardiology/American heart association task force on practice guidelines (committee to revise the 1995 guidelines for the evaluation and management of heart failure): developed in collaboration with the international society for heart and lung transplantation; endorsed by the heart failure society of America. *Circulation.*2001; 104:2996–3007.
25. Bardy GH, Lee KL, Mark DB et al. Amiodarone or an implantable cardioverter-defibrillator for congestive heart failure. *N Engl J Med*;2005; 352:225–237.
26. Cleland JG, Daubert JC, Erdmann E et al. The effect of cardiac resynchronization on morbidity and mortality in heart failure. *N Engl J Med.*2005; 352:1539–1549.
27. Dubin AM, Janousek J, Rhee E et al. Resynchronization therapy in pediatric and congenital heart disease patients: an international multicenter study. *J Am Coll Cardiol.* 2005;46:2277–2283.
28. Cecchin F, Frangini PA, Brown DW et al. Cardiac resynchronization therapy (and multisite pacing) in pediatrics and congenital heart disease: five years experience in a single institution. *J Cardiovasc Electrophysiol.*2008: 58–65.
29. Mee RB, Harada Y. Retraining of the left ventricle with a left ventricular assist device (Bio-Medicus) after the arterial switch operation. *J Thorac Cardiovasc Surg.*1991; 101:171–173.
30. Devaney EJ, Charpie JR, Ohye RG, Bove EL. Combined arterial switch and Senning operation for congenitally corrected transposition of the great arteries: patient selection and intermediate results. *J Thorac Cardiovasc Surg.*2003; 125:500–507.
31. Quinn DW, McGuirk SP, Metha C et al. The morphologic left ventricle that requires training by means of pulmonary artery banding before the double-switch procedure for congenitally corrected transposition of the great arteries is at risk of late dysfunction. *J Thorac Cardiovasc Surg.* 2008;135:1137–1144, 1144 e1–e2.
32. Poirier NC, Yu JH, Brizard CP, Mee RB. Long-term results of left ventricular reconditioning and anatomic correction for systemic right ventricular dysfunction after atrial switch procedures. *J Thorac Cardiovasc Surg.*2004; 127:975–981.
33. Blume ED, Naftel DC, Bastardi HJ, Duncan BW, Kirklin JK, Webber SA. Outcomes of children bridged to heart transplantation with ventricular assist devices: a multi-institutional study. *Circulation.*2006 ;113:2313–2319.
34. Shaddy RE, Webb G. Applying heart failure guidelines to adult congenital heart disease patients. *Expert Rev Cardiovasc Ther.*2008; 6:165–174.
35. Wernovsky G, Wypij D, Jonas RA et al. Postoperative course and hemodynamic profile after the arterial switch operation in neonates and infants. A comparison of low-flow cardiopulmonary bypass and circulatory arrest. *Circulation.*1995; 92:2226–2235.
36. Hutter PA, Bennink GB, Ay L, Raes IB, Hitchcock JF, Meijboom EJ. Influence of coronary anatomy and reimplantation on the long-term outcome of the arterial switch. *Eur J Cardiothorac Surg.*2000;18:207–213.
37. Pasquali SK, Hasselblad V, Li JS, Kong DF, Sanders SP. Coronary artery pattern and outcome of arterial switch operation for transposition of the great arteries: a meta-analysis. *Circulation.* 2002;106:2575–2580.
38. Schwartz ML, Jonas RA, Colan SD. Anomalous origin of left coronary artery from pulmonary artery: recovery of left ventricular function after dual coronary repair. *J Am Coll Cardiol.* 1997;30:547–553.
39. Braunwald E, Rutherford JD. Reversible ischemic left ventricular dysfunction: evidence for the "hibernating myocardium". *J Am Coll Cardiol.*1986; 8:1467–1470.

40. Rein AJ, Colan SD, Parness IA, Sanders SP. Regional and global left ventricular function in infants with anomalous origin of the left coronary artery from the pulmonary trunk: preoperative and postoperative assessment. *Circulation.*1987; 75:115–123.
41. del Nido PJ, Duncan BW, Mayer JE, Jr., Wessel DL, LaPierre RA, Jonas RA. Left ventricular assist device improves survival in children with left ventricular dysfunction after repair of anomalous origin of the left coronary artery from the pulmonary artery. *Ann Thorac Surg.* 1999;67:169–172.
42. Huebler M, Koster A, Redlin M et al. Repair of ALCAPA in a 4-kg patient followed by successful weaning and "off-pump" explantation of an apical venting pulsatile LVAD. *J Card Surg.*2005;20:261–263.
43. Kondo C, Nakazawa M, Momma K, Kusakabe K. Sympathetic denervation and reinnervation after arterial switch operation for complete transposition. *Circulation.*1998; 97:2414–2419.
44. Momose M, Kobayashi H, Ikegami H et al. Total and partial cardiac sympathetic denervation after surgical repair of ascending aortic aneurysm. *J Nucl Med.*2001; 42:1346–1350.
45. Gagliardi MG, Adorisio R, Crea F, Versacci P, Di Donato R, Sanders SP. Abnormal vasomotor function of the epicardial coronary arteries in children five to eight years after arterial switch operation: an angiographic and intracoronary Doppler flow wire study. *J Am Coll Cardiol.* 2005;46:1565–1572.
46. Basso C, Maron BJ, Corrado D, Thiene G. Clinical profile of congenital coronary artery anomalies with origin from the wrong aortic sinus leading to sudden death in young competitive athletes. *J Am Coll Cardiol.*2000; 35:1493–1501.
47. Daniels SR. Coronary risk factors in children. In: Allen HD, Driscoll DJ, Shaddy RE, Feltes T, eds. *Moss and Adams' Heart Disease in Infants, Children, and Adolescents, Including the Fetus and Young Adult.* 7th ed. Philadelphia, PA: Lippincott, Williams & Wilkins; 2007:1447–1479.
48. Brothers JA, Stephens P, Gaynor JW, Lorber R, Vricella LA, Paridon SM. Anomalous aortic origin of a coronary artery with an interarterial course: should family screening be routine? *J Am Coll Cardiol.*2008; 51:2062–2064.
49. Anderson JL, Adams CD, Antman EM et al. ACC/AHA 2007 guidelines for the management of patients with unstable angina/non-ST-Elevation myocardial infarction: a report of the American College of Cardiology/American Heart Association Task Force on Practice Guidelines (Writing Committee to Revise the 2002 Guidelines for the Management of Patients With Unstable Angina/Non-ST-Elevation Myocardial Infarction) developed in collaboration with the American College of Emergency Physicians, the Society for Cardiovascular Angiography and Interventions, and the Society of Thoracic Surgeons endorsed by the American Association of Cardiovascular and Pulmonary Rehabilitation and the Society for Academic Emergency Medicine. *J Am Coll Cardiol.*2007; 50:e1–e157.
50. Antman EM, Anbe DT, Armstrong PW et al. ACC/AHA guidelines for the management of patients with ST-elevation myocardial infarction-executive summary: a report of the American College of Cardiology/American Heart Association Task Force on Practice Guidelines (Writing Committee to Revise the 1999 Guidelines for the Management of Patients with Acute Myocardial Infarction). *Circulation.*2004; 110:588–636.
51. de Lemos JA, Blazing MA, Wiviott SD et al. Early intensive vs a delayed conservative simvastatin strategy in patients with acute coronary syndromes: phase Z of the A to Z trial. *JAMA.* 2004;292:1307–1316.
52. Cannon CP, Braunwald E, McCabe CH et al. Intensive versus moderate lipid lowering with statins after acute coronary syndromes. *N Engl J Med.*2004; 350:1495–1504.
53. Carabello BA. The current therapy for mitral regurgitation. *J Am Coll Cardiol.* 2008;52: 319–326.
54. Bonow RO, Carabello BA, Chatterjee K et al. Focused update incorporated into the ACC/AHA 2006 guidelines for the management of patients with valvular heart disease: a report of

the American College of Cardiology/American Heart Association Task Force on Practice Guidelines (Writing Committee to Revise the 1998 Guidelines for the Management of Patients With Valvular Heart Disease): endorsed by the Society of Cardiovascular Anesthesiologists, Society for Cardiovascular Angiography and Interventions, and Society of Thoracic Surgeons. *Circulation.*2008 ;118:e523–e661.

55. Krishnan US, Gersony WM, Berman-Rosenzweig E, Apfel HD. Late left ventricular function after surgery for children with chronic symptomatic mitral regurgitation. *Circulation* 1997;96: 4280–4285.
56. Leversha AM, Wilson NJ, Clarkson PM, Calder AL, Ramage MC, Neutze JM. Efficacy and dosage of enalapril in congenital and acquired heart disease. *Arch Dis Child.*1994; 70:35–39.
57. Mori Y, Nakazawa M, Tomimatsu H, Momma K. Long-term effect of angiotensin-converting enzyme inhibitor in volume overloaded heart during growth: a controlled pilot study. *J Am Coll Cardiol.*2000; 36:270–275.
58. Calabro R, Pisacane C, Pacileo G, Russo MG. Hemodynamic effects of a single oral dose of enalapril among children with asymptomatic chronic mitral regurgitation. *Am Heart J.* 1999;138:955–961.
59. Marcotte F, Honos GN, Walling AD et al. Effect of angiotensin-converting enzyme inhibitor therapy in mitral regurgitation with normal left ventricular function. *Can J Cardiol.* 1997;13:479–485.
60. Harris KM, Aeppli DM, Carey CF. Effects of angiotensin-converting enzyme inhibition on mitral regurgitation severity, left ventricular size, and functional capacity. *Am Heart J.* 2005;150:1106.
61. Dujardin KS, Enriquez-Sarano M, Bailey KR, Seward JB, Tajik AJ. Effect of losartan on degree of mitral regurgitation quantified by echocardiography. *Am J Cardiol.* 2001;87: 570–576.
62. Tsutsui H, Spinale FG, Nagatsu M et al. Effects of chronic beta-adrenergic blockade on the left ventricular and cardiocyte abnormalities of chronic canine mitral regurgitation. *J Clin Invest.* 1994;93:2639–2648.
63. Carabello BA. Aortic regurgitation. A lesion with similarities to both aortic stenosis and mitral regurgitation. *Circulation.*1990; 82:1051–1053.
64. Scognamiglio R, Rahimtoola SH, Fasoli G, Nistri S, Dalla Volta S. Nifedipine in asymptomatic patients with severe aortic regurgitation and normal left ventricular function. *N Engl J Med.*1994;331:689–694.
65. Sondergaard L, Aldershvile J, Hildebrandt P, Kelbaek H, Stahlberg F, Thomsen C. Vasodilatation with felodipine in chronic asymptomatic aortic regurgitation. *Am Heart J.* 2000;139:667–674.
66. Evangelista A, Tornos P, Sambola A, Permanyer-Miralda G, Soler-Soler J. Long-term vasodilator therapy in patients with severe aortic regurgitation. *N Engl J Med.* 2005;353: 1342–1349.
67. Carabello BA. Vasodilators in aortic regurgitation-where is the evidence of their effectiveness? *N Engl J Med.*2005; 353:1400–1402.
68. Lin M, Chiang HT, Lin SL et al. Vasodilator therapy in chronic asymptomatic aortic regurgitation: enalapril versus hydralazine therapy. *J Am Coll Cardiol.*1994; 24:1046–1053.
69. Alehan D, Ozkutlu S. Beneficial effects of 1-year captopril therapy in children with chronic aortic regurgitation who have no symptoms. *Am Heart J.*1998; 135:598–603.
70. Thompson LD, McElhinney DB, Culbertson CB et al. Perioperative administration of angiotensin converting enzyme inhibitors decreases the severity and duration of pleural effusions following bidirectional cavopulmonary anastomosis. *Cardiol Young.*2001; 11:195–200.
71. Kouatli AA, Garcia JA, Zellers TM, Weinstein EM, Mahony L. Enalapril does not enhance exercise capacity in patients after Fontan procedure. *Circulation.*1997; 96:1507–1512.
72. Ohuchi H, Hasegawa S, Yasuda K, Yamada O, Ono Y, Echigo S. Severely impaired cardiac autonomic nervous activity after the Fontan operation. *Circulation.*2001; 104:1513–1518

Heart Failure in Adults with Congenital HeartD isease

4

Konstantinos Dimopoulos, Georgios Giannakoulas,a nd Michael A. Gatzoulis

4.1
Heart Failure in Adults with Congenital Heart Disease

According to the latest guidelines for the diagnosis and treatment of heart failure by the American College of Cardiology/American Heart Association (ACC/AHA) and the European Society of Cardiology (ESC), heart failure is defined as a syndrome characterized by symptoms of exercise intolerance in the presence of any abnormality in the structure and/or function of the heart.[1,2] Almost all types of acquired or congenital heart disease, involving the myocardium, pericardium, endocardium, valves or great vessels, can thus ultimately lead to the development of heart failure and can be included in the spectrum of the heart failure syndrome.[3,4] Heart failure is the ultimate expression of the sequelae and complications, which adults with congenital heart disease (ACHD) often face, even after "successful" repair of their primary defect. In fact, even though surgical repair may appear to restore normal cardiac structure, more often than not subtle abnormalities of heart and/or extra-cardiac structures persist and may affect cardiac function. Multiple operations and arrhythmias may also cause cardiac dysfunction, causing signs and symptoms of heart failure.

4.1.1
The Prevalence of Heart Failure in Adults with Congenital Heart Disease

Exercise intolerance is the mainstay of heart failure. Exercise intolerance is common in this population affecting more than a third of patients in the Euro Heart Survey, a large registry of 4,110 ACHD patients across Europe (Fig. 4.1).[5] Patients with cyanotic lesions and those with a univentricular circulation tend to be those with the highest prevalence of exercise intolerance, whereas patients with aortic coarctation and Marfan's syndrome are the least impaired.[6,7] Within the cyanotic population, those with significant pulmonary arterial hypertension

K.D imopoulos (✉)
RoyalB romptonH ospital, SydneySt reet, London, SW36N P, UK
e-mail:k.dimopoulos @rbht.nhs.uk

R.E. Shaddy (ed.), *Heart Failure in Congenital Heart Disease*,
DOI: 10.1007/978-1-84996-480-7_4, © Springer-Verlag London Limited 2011

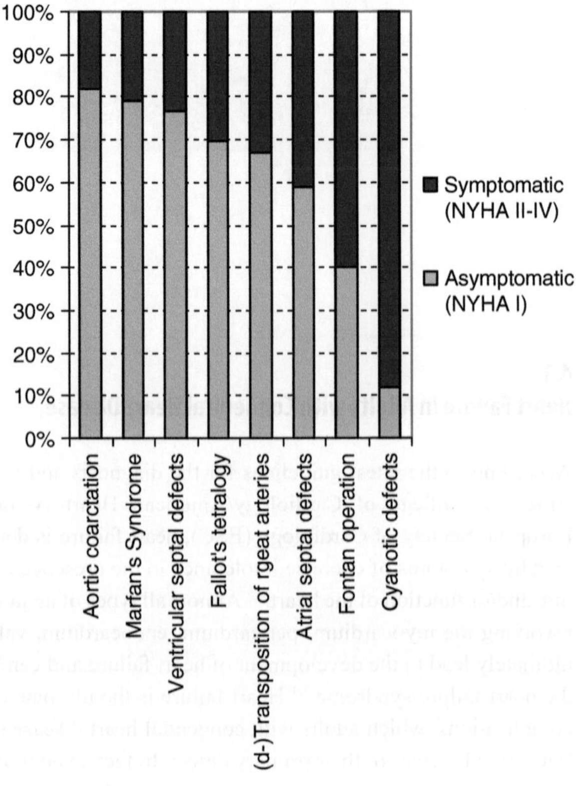

Fig.4.1 Percentageof symptomatic patients in various ACHD groups (Data from the Euro Heart survey in ACHD (n = 4110) [5])

(Eisenmenger syndrome) tend to be most severely limited.[7,8] Patients with the right ventricle in the systemic position, either as a result of congenitally corrected transposition of the great arteries or after atrial switch operation (Mustard or Senning procedure) for transposition of the great arteries also tend to become severely limited in their exercise capacity, especially after the third decade of life. As many as two thirds of patients with congenitally corrected transposition of the great arteries with significant associated defects and prior open heart surgery have congestive heart failure by age 45,[9] while in those with transposition of the great arteries who have undergone the Mustard procedure, 10% require hospital admission for congestive heart failure over a median follow up of 8 years.[10] Patients with univentricular circulation and a Fontan-type operation are also often limited in their exercise capacity, especially in the presence of ventricular dysfunction, atrioventricular valve regurgitation or a failing Fontan circuit. In a group of 188 patients with a systemic right ventricle or single ventricle, the frequency of heart failure was high (22% in transposition of the great arteries and intra-atrial baffles, 32% in corrected transposition of the great arteries and 40% in Fontan-palliated patients).[11] However, even patients with "simple" native lesions such as atrial septal defects (ASDs) often present with signs and symptoms of heart failure, even though often at a later stage (after the fifth to sixth decade of life).[12]

4.2 Quantification and Follow-up of Exercise Intolerance

4.2.1 Subjective Quantification

The first step for assessing exercise intolerance is quantification of its severity. This can be achieved either by subjective (describing patients' perception of their limitation) or objective means. The most commonly used classification for quantifying subjective limitation in ACHD is the New York Heart Association (NYHA) classification (Table 4.1). This scale is preferred as it is familiar to adult cardiologists and is simple and easy to apply. When compared to objective measures of exercise capacity, the NYHA classification is able to stratify ACHD patients according to their exercise capacity, but overall tends to underestimate their degree of impairment. In fact, many asymptomatic (NYHA I) ACHD patients have dramatically lower objective exercise capacity compared to normal controls, which is similar to that of much older patients with acquired heart failure.[7] It appears in fact that ACHD patients tend to be less aware of their exercise limitation, as this has occurred over several decades rather than abruptly as occurs in acquire heart failure. This apparent unawareness of significant exercise limitation in many ACHD patients may impact on the timing and type of therapeutic interventions, possibly supporting a "sooner rather than

Table4. 1 New York Class Association and the Ability Index Classifications

Class	New York Class Association	Abilityi ndex
1.	Patients have cardiac disease but without the resulting limitations of physical activity. Ordinary physical activity does not cause undue fatigue, palpitation, dyspnea, or anginal pain	Normal life, full time work or school, can manage pregnancy
2.	Patients have cardiac disease resulting in slight limitation of physical activity. They are comfortable at rest. Ordinary physical activity results in fatigue, palpitation, dyspnea, or anginal pain	Able to do part time work, life modified by symptoms
3.	Patients have cardiac disease resulting in marked limitation of physical activity. They are comfortable at rest. Less than ordinary physical activity causes fatigue, palpitation, dyspnea, or anginal pain	Unable to work, noticeable limitation of activities
4.	Patients have cardiac disease resulting in inability to carry on any physical activity without discomfort. Symptoms of cardiac insufficiency or of the anginal syndrome may be present even at rest. If any physical activity is undertaken, discomfort is increased	Extreme limitation, dependent, almost housebound

later" approach.[13] In particular, patients with right-sided lesions such as patients with severe pulmonary regurgitation after repair of Fallot's tetralogy, tend to remain asymptomatic or very mildly symptomatic for long, even in the presence of significant right ventricular dilation and dysfunction.[14] It is, thus, important that objective means of assessment such as cardiopulmonary exercise testing be used for the routine clinical assessment of ACHD patients and aid in the decision making when considering elective surgery.

NYHA classification cannot be used as health-related quality of life score. Scores specifically developed for the assessment of the quality of life of patients with ACHD are available, such as the Ability Index (Table 4.1).[15] Their use has, nevertheless, been limited by scarce familiarity within the adult cardiology environment and the limited data on their reliability and validity.

4.2.2 Objective Quantification

4.2.2.1 Cardiopulmonary Exercise Testing

The best method for quantifying exercise tolerance in health (athletes) and disease is cardiopulmonary exercise testing. It is a powerful tool for the objective assessment of the cardiovascular, respiratory and muscular systems and has become part of the routine clinical assessment of ACHD patients. Incremental (ramp) protocols are used to assess functional and prognostic indices such as the peak oxygen consumption (peak VO_2), the VE/VCO_2 slope (the slope of the regression line between ventilation and VCO_2), the anaerobic threshold and the heart rate and blood pressure response.

Peak VO_2 is the highest value of oxygen uptake recorded during maximal exercise testing and approximates the maximal aerobic power of an individual, i.e. the upper limit of oxygen utilization by the body (Fig. 4.2). It is usually expressed in mL/kg/min and reflects the functional status of the pulmonary, cardiovascular and muscular systems. In fact, during steady state, oxygen uptake from the lungs reflects the amount of oxygen consumed by the cells in the periphery. Peak VO_2 is the most reported exercise parameter because it is simple to interpret and carries prognostic power both in acquired heart failure and ACHD.[7] However, peak VO_2 can only be reliably estimated from maximal exercise tests and is limited by the ability and determination of a patient to exercise to exhaustion. Moreover, it can be prone to technical error/artifacts as it is derived from measurements recorded only during the last minute of exercise (peak).

Cardiopulmonary exercise testing in a large cohort of ACHD patients demonstrated that average peak VO_2 was depressed in all ACHD subgroups compared to healthy subjects of similar age and varied according to underlying anatomy (Fig. 4.3).[7] Peak VO_2 was significantly depressed even in asymptomatic ACHD patients (Fig. 4.4). Patients with Eisenmenger physiology and complex anatomy (univentricular hearts with protected pulmonary circulation) had the lowest average peak VO_2 values (11.5 and 14.6 mL/kg/min respectively). Gender, body mass index, cyanosis, pulmonary arterial hypertension, forced expiratory volume, and peak heart rate were independent predictors of peak VO_2 in this population.

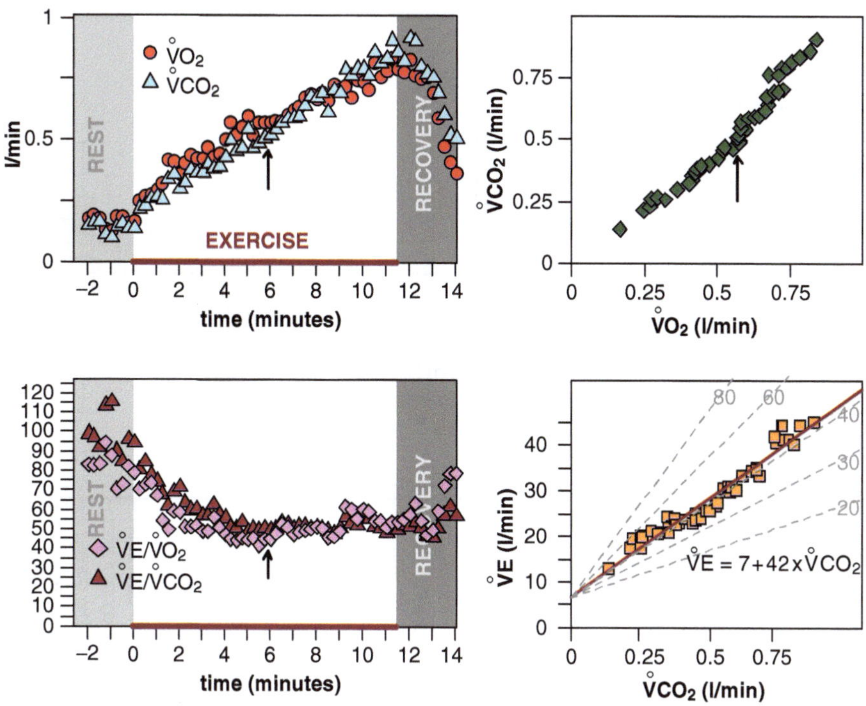

Fig. 4.2 Example of cardiopulmonary exercise testing in a moderately symptomatic (NYHA class III) patient after a Fontan-type operation. The patient exercised for 11.5 min and reached respiratory exchange ratio of 1.1. No drop in arterial oxygen saturation was recorded. Peak VO_2 was 21.6 mL/kg/min, which is 55% of predicted (*upper left panel*). VE/VCO_2 slope was significantly increased (43.6) suggesting pulmonary hypoperfusion and ventilation/perfusion mismatch (*lower right panel*). Anaerobic threshold was 14.1 mL/kg/min (*upper right panel*)

Patients with permanent pacemakers, on beta-blocker therapy and those not in sinus rhythm also had lower peak VO_2. Exercise capacity in ACHD patients was independent of resting cardiac function as with acquired heart failure.[16] Peak VO_2 is an independent predictor of the combined endpoint of death or hospitalization in ACHD at a median follow-up of 304 days; patients with a peak $VO_2 < 15.5$ mL/kg/min had a threefold increased risk of death.[7] Peak VO_2 is also related to the frequency and duration of hospitalization, even after accounting for NYHA class, age, age at surgery and gender. Peak circulatory power expressed as peak exercise oxygen uptake multiplied by peak mean arterial blood pressure has also been shown to be a strong predictor of adverse outcome in ACHD.[17]

The anaerobic threshold is the level of VO_2 beyond which aerobic metabolism is substantially supplemented by anaerobic processes.[18,19] Above the anaerobic threshold, lactate starts to accumulate and is buffered by plasma bicarbonate, resulting in an increase in CO_2 production (VCO_2). Anaerobic threshold can be identified through observation of the VCO_2 versus VO_2 relation, or by observing the ventilation (VE)/VO_2 ratio over time.[18,19] The anaerobic threshold has an obvious pathophysiologic significance as it is the point at

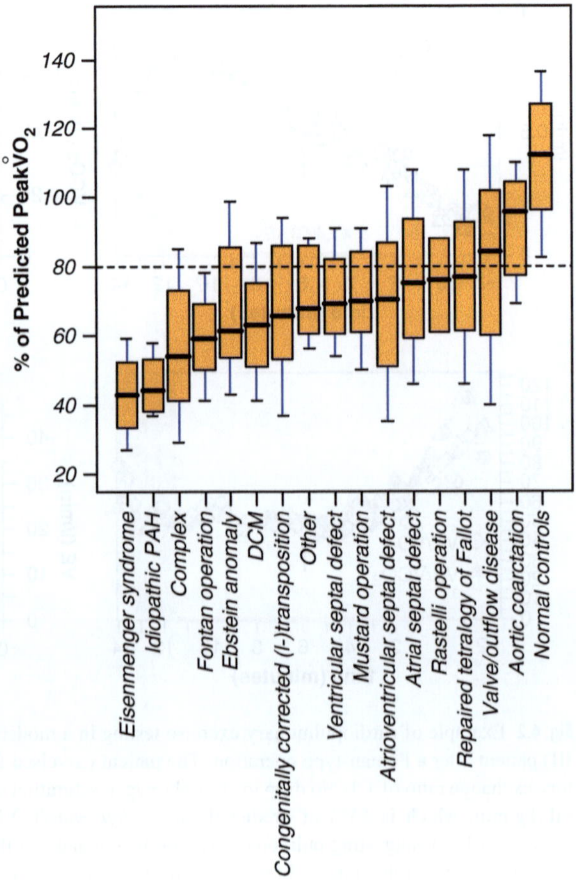

Fig. 4.3 Peak VO_2 in various types of ACHD and normal controls. Boxplots depict median and interquartile range. Whiskers depict range. Exercise capacity is significantly lower compared to normal controls in all ACHD groups and is lowest in patients with Eisenmenger syndrome and or complex/univentricular anatomy. A group of patients with idiopathic pulmonary hypertension is also shown for comparison (Data from[8])

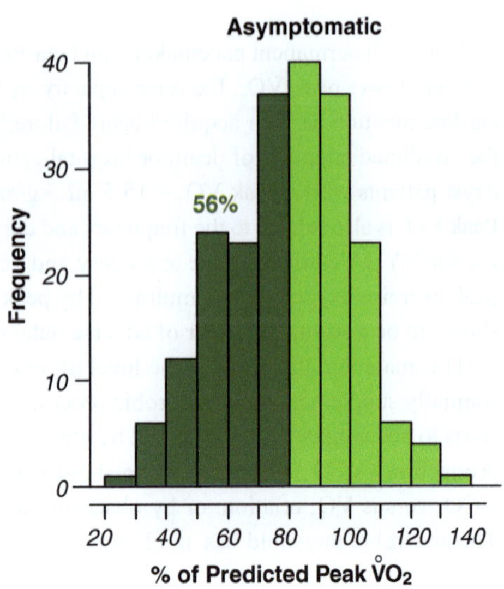

Fig. 4. 4 Distribution of peak VO_2 in asymptomatic ACHD patients. In this asymptomatic group, 50–60% of patients have an abnormal peak VO_2 (less than 80% of predicted), suggesting that patients underestimate their degree of exercise intolerance (Data from[8])

which aerobic metabolism is unable to sustain energy requirement. It also carries important prognostic information in acquired heart failure and ACHD.[7,20–22]

The VE/VCO$_2$ slope is an exercise parameter that is independent of maximal exertion (Fig. 4.2). It is a simplification of the complex relationship between ventilation and CO$_2$ production. It is thought to reflect pulmonary perfusion and the degree of physiological dead space and ventilation/perfusion mismatch, as well as enhanced ventilatory reflex sensitivity. It is easy to calculate, reproducible and a marker of exercise intolerance strongly related to peak VO$_2$. The VE/VCO$_2$ slope carries important physiological and prognostic information.[8]

High values of VE/VCO$_2$ slope compared to normal controls were also encountered in major ACHD subgroups.[8] Patients with Eisenmenger physiology were found to have the most disproportionately high VE/VCO$_2$ slopes (mean 71.2), whereas patients with aortic coarctation had the lowest mean VE/VCO$_2$ slope (29.4) (Fig. 4.5). Cyanosis had a significant impact on the ventilatory response to exercise and was the strongest independent predictor of the VE/VCO$_2$ slope in this cohort. A linear relation between VE/VCO$_2$ slope and NYHA class was observed, suggesting a link between the ventilatory response to exercise

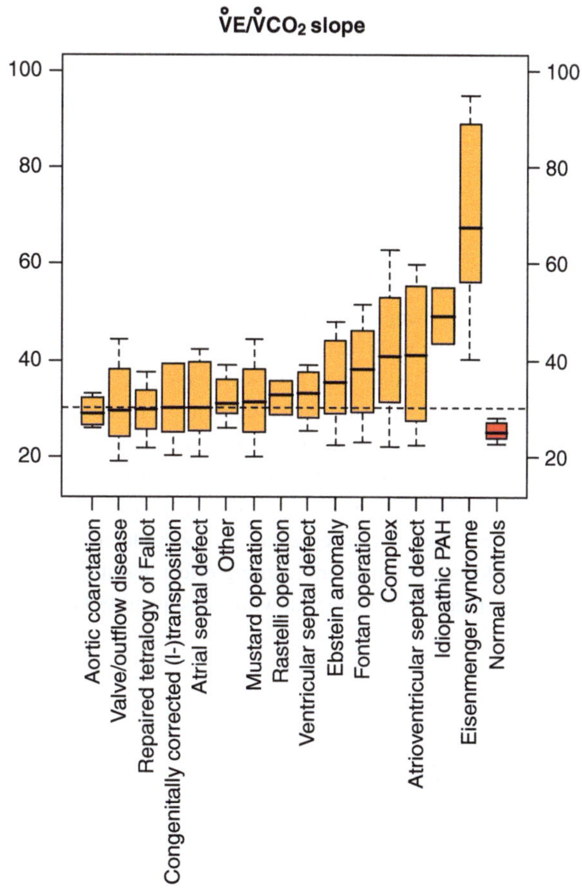

Fig. 4.5 Distribution of VE/VCO$_2$ slope values in ACHD patients. The VE/VCO$_2$ slope is significantly higher in most ACHD groups compared to normal controls and highest in the cyanotic population (Data from[8])

and the occurrence of symptoms. Nevertheless, the VE/VCO_2 slope was, like in the case of peak VO_2, significantly raised even amongst asymptomatic patients, further underscoring the importance of objective assessment of exercise capacity in ACHD. A VE/VCO_2 slope of 38 or above is an adverse prognostic marker in non-cyanotic ACHD patients, associated with a tenfold increase in the risk of death within 2 years. VE/VCO_2 slope has been found to be improved after pulmonary valve replacement in patients with tetralogy of Fallot.[23] Those patients who were younger than 17.5 years old, at the time of pulmonary valve replacement, were more likely to have a normal VE/VCO_2 slope 1 year after surgery.

4.2.2.2
Six-Minute Walk Test

A simpler means of objectively assessing exercise capacity is the 6-minute walk test. It is a submaximal timed distance exercise test, easy to perform and reflects ordinary daily activities. The main response variable is the distance, which individuals cover at their own pace in 6 min. A normal subject of age 40 years is normally able to cover approximately 600 m, decreasing by 50 m per decade. Oxygen saturations by portable pulse oximetry and perceived exertion through semiquantitative means such as the Borg scale can also be recorded.

The six minute walk test is best used in significantly impaired patients, since in healthy and mildly impaired individuals it is a submaximal test. In fact, 6-minute walk test distance correlates well with peak VO_2 in highly symptomatic patients. A cut-off value of 450 m in the 6-minute walk test allows a semiquantitative classification in analogy to Grade C in the classification suggested of Weber for cardiopulmonary exercise testing (peak VO_2 between 10 to 16 mL/min/kg), and to a level of brain natriuretic peptide in the plasma of less or more than 100 picograms per milliliter.[24,25]

The 6 minute walk test is thought to be more sensitive to changes following intervention compared to peak VO_2. It is nowadays used to assess the response to advanced therapies in patients with pulmonary hypertension and is the only test approved by the U.S. Food and Drug Administration (FDA) as an endpoint for prospective clinical trials in this population. Its use in mildly symptomatic patients is, nevertheless, limited by a "ceiling effect," which could mask improvement after intervention. Adequate standardization of the protocol used is also essential for guaranteeing reproducibility and comparability of repeated tests. An important learning effect has also been described and should be kept in mind when comparing the first with subsequent tests.

4.3
Mechanisms of Heart Failure in ACHD

Exercise intolerance can occur in ACHD through a variety of mechanisms, both cardiac ande xtracardiac(Fig. 4.6).

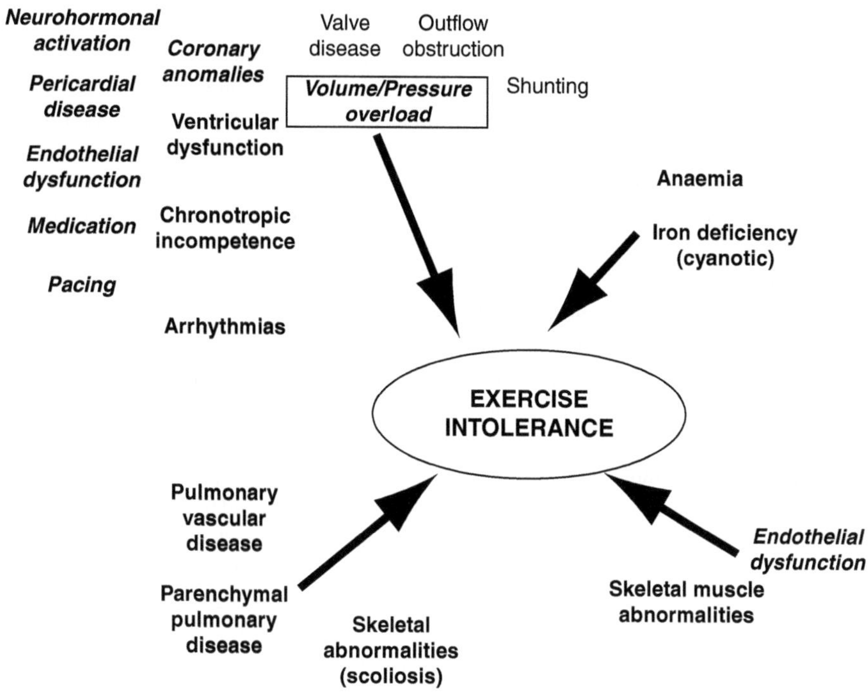

Fig. 4.6 Mechanisms of exercise intolerance in ACHD patients. Exercise intolerance in ACHD is multifactorial and can be due to a variety of cardiac and non-cardiac causes

4.3.1 Cardiac Causes of Exercise Intolerance in ACHD

4.3.1.1 Ventricular Dysfunction

Cardiac dysfunction is the most obvious cause of exercise intolerance and heart failure in ACHD. A reduction in cardiac output may occur through a reduction in ventricular function (reduced stroke volume) or through inability to increase heart rate to meet demands. Myocardial dysfunction is common in ACHD and can be caused by ventricular overload, myocardial ischemia and pericardial disease. It can also occur through the effects of medication, permanent pacing, endothelial and neurohormonal activation.

Most types of congenital cardiac defects can result in hemodynamic overload of one or both ventricles due to obstructive or regurgitant lesions, shunting, pulmonary or systemic hypertension. This overload is, by definition in ACHD, long-standing, and can over time lead to severe ventricular dysfunction. Significant systemic ventricular dysfunction is found 10–30 years after surgery in patients after atrial repair of (d-) transposition of the great arteries, corrected (l-) transposition of the great arteries, and patients with Fontan-type circulation. Right ventricular systolic dysfunction may develop with time in patients with significant volume overload such as those with large ASDs or patients with tetralogy of Fallot and severe pulmonary regurgitation. Left ventricular dysfunction can be the result of congenital aortic regurgitation or stenosis, aortic coarctation, and significant left atrioventricular valve regurgitation in patients with atrioventricular septal defects. Ventricular dysfunction can also result from repeated cardiac surgery and protracted cardiopulmonary by-pass, especially in previous eras when myocardial protection and cardioplegia may have been suboptimal. Repeat or extensive ventriculotomies and patch augmentation of the right ventricular outflow tract do also contribute to ventricular dysfunction. Ventricular dysfunction can also occur in patients with pericardial disease (congenital absence of pericardium or constrictive pericarditis related to previous surgery).

Suboptimal myocardial perfusion may also contribute to the development of ventricular dysfunction in ACHD. Myocardial infarction can occur in patients with anomalous origin of the left coronary artery from the pulmonary artery and lead to left ventricular dilation and dysfunction. An anomalous left coronary artery may be severed during right ventricular outflow tract patching to repair tetralogy of Fallot, leading to apical aneurysm formation, ventricular tachycardia, heart failure and death. Reversible and fixed perfusion defects with concordant regional wall motion abnormalities have been documented in patients after atrial or arterial switch repair for transposition of the great arteries and are thought to affect ventricular function. A great number of ACHD patients are born with a coronary circulation which, by conventional criteria, would be classified as anomalous. Whether these abnormalities in the origin and distribution of the coronary circulation seen in ACHD can affect ventricular function long-term, remains unknown.

Ventricular dysfunction may also be triggered or exacerbated by arrhythmias, permanent pacing and medication. ACHD patients have an increased propensity to arrhythmias due to intrinsic abnormalities of the conduction system, long-standing hemodynamic overload and scarring from reparative or palliative surgery. Arrhythmias in ACHD patients can lead to significant hemodynamic compromise, especially in the presence of myocardial dysfunction and can become life-threatening, especially when fast or ventricular in origin. Even relatively slow supraventricular tachycardias may, however, cause a reduction in cardiac output and exercise capacity through loss of atrioventricular synchrony, especially when long-standing.

Often left ventricular dysfunction occurs in ACHD patients with right-sided lesions, which may be difficult to explain. Ventricular–ventricular interaction is not uncommon in ACHD, with right-sided lesions often affecting the left ventricle and vice-versa. Significant ventricular interaction is most pronounced in patients with Ebstein's anomaly, in whom the left ventricle typically appears small, underfilled and hypokinetic, almost "compressed" by the dilated right ventricular cavity. In other entities such as patients with restrictive ventricular septal defects and left ventricular dysfunction, this phenomenon may be more difficult to explain and may suggest an intrinsic predisposition to myocardial dysfunction and heart failure.

Diastolic dysfunction is also an important component of ACHD and can affect exercise capacity and ventricular response to overload. Restrictive right ventricular filling has been described in up to 50% of patients with tetralogy of Fallot late after repair and relates to a decreased predisposition to right ventricular dilation in the presence of significant pulmonary regurgitation.[26] However, right ventricular restriction in tetralogy appears to adversely affect right ventricular performance, and prolong the postoperative course in the immediate postoperative period.[26] The Holt-Oram syndrome was also found to be associated with abnormal left ventricular diastolic properties, which, from an animal model, may be related to abnormal regulation of SERCA2 and calcium handling due to Tbx5 haploinsufficiency.[27]

Acquired disease superimposed on the congenitally abnormal heart may also cause deterioration of myocardial dysfunction. Infective endocarditis, systemic hypertension, coronary atherosclerosis, myocarditis, alcohol or other substance abuse (i.e. cocaine) and diabetes mellitus may all trigger or aggravate myocardial dysfunction in ACHD. Infective endocarditis, in particular, even though relatively uncommon, can have devastating short and long-term effects on ACHD patients, who are at particularly high risk, in view of residual hemodynamic lesions and prosthetic material used.

The prevalence of significant coronary artery disease does not appear to be increased in ACHD patients,[28] however, as this population is ageing, coronary artery disease should always be suspected when ventricular dysfunction is encountered and traditional cardiovascular risk factors for coronary atherosclerosis should be addressed and be modified.

4.3.1.2 Chronotropic Incompetence

The chronotropic response to exercise is a major contributor to the increase in cardiac output, more so than the increase in myocardial contractility. Chronotropic incompetence may be defined as the inability to increase heart rate appropriate to the degree of effort and metabolic demands. Chronotropic incompetence is common in ACHD, encountered in 62% of ACHD patients in one series, and can be due to intrinsic abnormalities of the conduction system or iatrogenic.[29] Chronotropic incompetence in the ACHD population is related to the severity of exercise intolerance, plasma natriuretic peptide levels and peak oxygen uptake.[30] Furthermore, chronotropic incompetence is a strong predictor of mortality in ACHD patients, especially those with "complex" lesions, Fontan-type surgery and repaired tetralogy of Fallot.[29,31,32]

Medication such as beta-blockers, calcium antagonists and antiarrhythmics can have significant negative inotropic and chronotropic effects and thus may affect ventricular performance and exercise capacity. ACHD patients on beta-blockers tend to achieve a lower peak heart rate and a lower peak VO_2 during maximal exercise testing.[7] Medication can also unmask latent conduction system disease and lead to sinus node dysfunction, atrioventricular block or chronotropic incompetence.

Permanent pacing can also affect cardiac output through chronotropic incompetence and ventricular dysfunction. ACHD patients with a permanent pacemaker were, in fact, found to have significantly lower peak heart rate and a trend towards lower peak VO_2 compared to those without. Pacemaker therapy is often required in ACHD for atrioventricular block, common in patients with atrioventricular septal defects or corrected transposition of the great arteries and, in the past, immediately after surgical repair of a ventricular septal defect or muscle bundle resection. Sinus node dysfunction requiring permanent pacing is also common after Fontan operation or atrial switch repair for complete transposition of the great arteries. Dual-chamber pacemakers are most commonly used to avoid atrioventricular asynchrony, but this is not always possible in patients with complex anatomy. Moreover, despite advances in rate-responsive pacemakers, rate responsiveness at higher levels of exercise in younger patients may be inadequate to produce a sufficient increase in cardiac output. Right ventricular pacing can also cause ventricular asynchrony and, in the non-congenital population, has been shown to cause long-term left ventricular dysfunction and reduced exercise capacity. The development of sophisticated pacing technologies that encourage more intrinsic conduction, thus minimizing ventricular pacing, holds promise for ACHD patients.[32]

4.3.2 Extracardiac Causes of Exercise Intolerance in ACHD

4.3.2.1 Lung Disease, Pulmonary Arterial Hypertension and Cyanosis

Parenchymal and vascular lung disease are important contributors to exercise intolerance in ACHD. Subnormal forced vital capacity affects exercise capacity and has been reported in patients with Ebstein's anomaly, tetralogy of Fallot, corrected transposition of the great arteries, after the Fontan operation and after atrial repair for d-transposition of the great arteries, and even in patients with ASDs. Percentage of FEV1 has, in fact, been shown to be a powerful predictor of exercise capacity in the ACHD population.[7] Prior surgery with lung scarring, atelectasis, chest deformities, diaphragmatic palsy, pulmonary vascular disease with loss of distensibility of peripheral arteries and significant cardiomegaly are possible mechanisms for the abnormal pulmonary function observed in ACHD.

4.3.2.2 Pulmonary Arterial Hypertension and Cyanosis

Patients with Eisenmenger physiology are by far the most symptomatic amongst patients with pulmonary arterial hypertension associated with congenital heart disease, with 84% complaining of major exercise intolerance by age 28, suggesting a detrimental effect of cyanosis and pulmonary arterial hypertension. Patients with complex univentricular anatomy are also highly symptomatic, especially in the presence of significant cyanosis, and this is confirmed by objective data. Cyanosis and pulmonary arterial hypertension significantly affect exercise capacity and the ventilatory response to exercise. In these patients, an increase in cardiac output is obtained through intracardiac right-to-left shunting, at the expense of further systemic desaturation.

Oxygen uptake fails to increase at the onset of exercise due to the inability of the patient to sufficiently increase pulmonary blood flow. Ventilation increases abruptly and excessively resulting in alveolar hyperventilation, a rise in VCO_2 and a drop in VO_2.

While ventilation is increased throughout exercise, high values of the VE/VCO_2 slope in cyanotic patients suggest that ventilatory efficiency is significantly decreased. Pulmonary hypoperfusion, an increase in physiological dead-space through right-to-left shunting and enhanced ventilatory reflex sensitivity are potential mechanisms contributing to the ventilatory inefficiency and the failure to meet oxygen requirements in ACHD patients with cyanosis and pulmonary arterial hypertension.

The effect of cyanosis on exercise capacity and ventilation is difficult to distinguish from that of pulmonary arterial hypertension. Significant ventilatory inefficiency and a hyperventilatory response to exercise have also been described in patients with idiopathic pulmonary arterial hypertension in the absence of right-to-left shunting. The VE/VCO_2 slope of patients with significant pulmonary arterial hypertension and cyanosis is significantly higher than those without cyanosis, suggesting that cyanosis has an additive effect on ventilation, over that of pulmonary arterial hypertension. Moreover, Fontan patients with cyanosis have higher VE/VCO_2 slopes compared to those without, suggesting a significant effect of cyanosis on ventilation even in the absence of pulmonary arterial hypertension. Despite being "inefficient" and likely contributing to the early onset of dyspnea, the exaggerated ventilatory response to exercise in cyanotic ACHD patients appears appropriate from a "chemical" point of view as it succeeds in maintaining near-normal arterial PCO_2 and pH levels in the systemic circulation despite significant right-to-left shunting, at least during mild-to-moderate exertion.[4,22]

4.3.2.3 Anemia and Iron-Deficiency

Anemia relates to exercise capacity in acquired heart failure and is a predictor of outcome. Anemia results in reduced oxygen carrying capacity and a premature shift to anaerobic metabolism during exercise and can precipitate heart failure by affecting myocardial function and volume overload. Anemia in ACHD can occur as a complication of chronic anticoagulation, surgery or intervention, hemolysis due to prosthetic valves, intracardiac patches or endocarditis, or hemoptysis in patients with severe pulmonary arterial hypertension. Moreover, anemia can occur due to chronic renal failure or as the anemia of chronic disease.

Anemia as conventionally defined is rare in cyanotic patients. Chronic hypoxia results in an increase in erythropoietin production and an isolated rise in the red blood cell count (secondary erythrocytosis) which augments the amount of oxygen delivered to the tissues. "Relative anemia" i.e. inadequate rise in hemoglobin levels despite chronic cyanosis can, nevertheless, occur as a result of iron deficiency and may have detrimental effects on exercise capacity and symptoms, including an increased risk of transient ischemic attacks and stroke. However, no universally accepted algorithm for the calculation of "appropriate" hemoglobin levels exists. In general, secondary erythrocytosis is inversely related to severity of cyanosis in iron replete patients and the diagnosis of relative anemia in this setting should be based on serum ferritin and transferrin saturation levels.[33]

4.4 Systemic Manifestations of the Heart Failure Syndrome in ACHD

The clinical syndrome of heart failure has important systemic manifestations, which define its natural history and are the target of modern therapies. Neurohormonal activation, chemoreflex and peripheral ergoreflex activation as well as organ failure, such as renal and hepatic dysfunction, are well described complications of acquired heart failure and affect the outcome of these patients. Neurohormonal and cytokine activation have also been described in ACHD patients, with elevated atrial natriuretic peptide, B-type natriuretic peptide, endothelin-1, renin, aldosterone and norepinephrine reported across a wide spectrum of congenital lesions and correlating with worsening NYHA class and ventricular function.[34,35] Neurohormonal activation has also been described in asymptomatic patients years after surgical repair of even relatively simple lesions.

Deranged cardiac autonomic nervous activity, a marker of adverse outcome in chronic heart failure and ischemic heart disease, is also common in ACHD patients late after repair of tetralogy of Fallot and in patients after Fontan-type circulation.[36,37] Impaired autonomic nervous activity plays a contributory role in higher incidence of tachyarrhythmia during pregnancy in patients with repaired ACHD.[38,39] Autonomic dysfunction in ACHD is likely the result of a chronic low cardiac output state, but may also be secondary to damage of cardiac innervation during surgery and the effects of cardiopulmonary bypass. Autonomic indices are related to hemodynamic status, prior history of arrhythmias and markers of ventricular tachycardia or sudden cardiac death, suggesting a possible prognostic impact of autonomic derangement in ACHD. Impaired cardiac autonomic nervous activity was associated with an increased risk of sudden cardiac death in a small study of 43 ACHD patients.[40]

Skeletal muscle wasting is common in heart failure and can become severe, with profound effects on blood flow to the limbs.[41,42] Histologic and metabolic abnormalities (changes in fiber type content and fiber dimension, mitochondrial function, oxidative processes) result in a premature shift to anaerobic metabolism, early fatigability and reduction in strength.[43–45] Muscle ergoreceptors located in the exercising skeletal muscle sense the metabolic changes occurring in the muscle fibers mediating sympathetic activation and vasoconstriction. Overactivity of the muscle ergoreflex system in heart failure may lead to progressive neurohormonal activation and mediate an increased ventilatory response leading to the premature occurrence of dyspnea and fatigue.[46–48] Increased chemoreflex sensitivity is also present in heart failure, likely due to low cardiac output and the potentiating effect on chemosensitivity of catecholamines.

Suggestion of peripheral metaboreflex (ergoreflex) hypersensitivity and chemoreflex activation has been provided by small studies.[49,50] Vonder Muhll et al. also demonstrated that one out of ten ACHD patients have evidence of cachexia, more prevalent in patients with univentricular circulation and those with cyanosis.[51] Brassard et al. also demonstrated an improvement in ergoreflex activity after an 8-week training program in patients with Fontan circulation.[49] In fact, exercise training increases blood flow to the legs and improves ventilatory control in chronic heart failure, as well as produces a partial reversal of histologic and metabolic abnormalities in the skeletal muscles and a reduction in muscle wasting.[52–55] Chemoreflex and ergoreflex activation are likely to affect the ventilatory response to exercise and may explain the early occurrence of dyspnea in ACHD patients.[56,57]

Cytokine activation is an important component of the heart failure syndrome, especially in more advanced stages, and is a strong prognostic marker in this setting. Cytokine activation has also been described in ACHD patients. Sharma et al. reported high levels of tumor necrosis factor (TNF) in ACHD patients, which correlated well with functional class.[58] Cytokines levels were particularly high in cyanotic patients and those with peripheral edema. A significant correlation between levels of TNF receptor-1 and systemic ventricular dysfunction was also described.

Endothelial dysfunction is thought to play an important role in the pathophysiology of acquired heart failure. It is thought to have a detrimental effect on myocardial and skeletal muscle function and be involved in the development of heart failure and exercise intolerance. It correlates with functional impairment and natriuretic peptide levels, improves with appropriate therapy and is a predictor of outcome in patients with advanced heart failure. Evidence of endothelial dysfunction in congenital heart disease is available for Fontan patients and for cyanotic ACHD patients, in whom it appears to result from a reduced production or release of nitric oxide despite the hemoconcentration and increase in shear stress.[59] Eisenmenger patients also exhibit reduced circulating endothelial progenitor cells and raised levels of inflammatory mediators such as immune inflammatory markers, cGMP, stable nitric oxide oxidation products, and asymmetric dimethylarginine.[60]

Renal dysfunction is common in patients with acquired heart failure and the term "cardiorenal syndrome" is nowadays used to define a state of advanced cardiorenal dysregulation. ACHD patients, even though younger than those with acquired heart failure, also have a high prevalence of impaired renal function with moderate or severe dysfunction present in one out of five patients.[61] Renal dysfunction in ACHD is likely to be due to low cardiac output state with decreased kidney perfusion, activation of sympathetic nervous system leading to arterial vasoconstriction and activation of the renin-angiotensin-aldosterone system. Cyanotic patients are at highest risk of developing renal dysfunction, suggesting a detrimental effect of chronic hypoxia and, perhaps, hyperviscosity on the kidney. Patients with moderate to severe renal dysfunction had a threefold increased risk of death.

Hypotonic hyponatremia is typical of patients with congestive heart failure, especially those requiring treatment with diuretics, and is a strong prognostic marker in this population and a criterion for transplantation. Hyponatremia has also been found to be common in ACHD patients, affecting one out of seven, and is a predictor of outcome independent of renal dysfunction and use of diuretics.[62]

4.5 Treatment

4.5.1 Treatment of Target Hemodynamic Lesions and Correctable Abnormalities

Cardiac dysfunction is a major determinant of exercise intolerance in ACHD and cardiac hemodynamic lesions should be the first target in an effort to improve exercise capacity. Potential therapeutic options include surgical or interventional relief of obstructive lesions, repair of valve abnormalities and elimination or reduction of shunts.[4,63] Improvement in symptoms has been reported after interventions such as Fontan-type operations, tetralogy of Fallot repair, relief of congenital aortic stenosis and percutaneous closure of ASD.[64–68] Correction of such lesions may affect not only the functional capacity, but also the longer-term outcome for these patients.[69] Other reversible causes of exercise intolerance and ventricular dysfunction, such as ischemic heart disease, anemia and parenchymal pulmonary disease should be sought and treated, when possible.

4.5.2 Counteracting Neurohormonal Activation

Medical treatment of chronic heart failure is nowadays based on counteracting neurohormonal activation with drugs such as beta-adrenergic receptor blockers, angiotensin converting enzyme (ACE) inhibitors, angiotensin receptor blockers and spironolactone, improving not just hemodynamics but also prognosis. Such drugs are increasingly being used in ACHD on the basis of similarities in pathophysiology between ACHD and acquired heart failure.[70] This approach is, however, arbitrary, as it is not based on solid scientific evidence and ignores important differences between the two conditions and the unique characteristics of individual congenital heart defects, which may influence drug dosage, tolerability and effectiveness.[4,8,33,61,71] Despite numerous attempts, no hard evidence of the beneficial effects of such medication on stable compensated ACHD patients is yet available (Table 4.2).[72–79] Published trials are mostly single center studies with a sample size significantly smaller compared to similar trials in acquired heart disease.

Two studies in pediatric Fontan patients showed no beneficial effect of ACE inhibitors.[73,80] ACE inhibitors have been used in patients after atrial switch for transposition of great arteries showing no significant improvement in exercise capacity or right ventricular function,[76,81] while losartan, an angiotensin receptor blocker, resulted in a decrease in tricuspid regurgitation and an improvement in exercise time.[74] ACE inhibitors were thought to present a risk to cyanotic patients due to a potential increase in right-to-left shunting caused by the drop in left ventricular afterload. However, a small retrospective report on ten patients showed no adverse effects of ACE inhibition (captopril and enalapril) on blood pressure and oxygen saturation and an improvement in symptomatic status and quality of life at 1 year.[82] A study of ACE inhibition in patients with repaired tetralogy of Fallot and significant pulmonary regurgitation failed to show any significant effect of ramipril on right ventricular function.[75]

Beta blockers in infants with heart failure secondary to left-to-right shunting at the ventricular level resulted in an improvement in clinical status and neurohormonal levels.[83] Beta blockers in ACHD patients after aortic valve replacement resulted in a reduction in left ventricular size.[84] A pilot study of eight patients after atrial repair for d-transposition of the great arteries or corrected transposition of the great arteries and chronic heart failure showed that carvedilol administration may be safe and was associated with positive right ventricular remodeling as well as improved exercise duration.[85] Other reports, however, showed no beneficial effects of bisoprolol on the clinical status and neurohormonal levels of patients with tetralogy of Fallot.[78] A multicenter study by Shaddy et al. in pediatric and adolescents patients ($n = 161$), showed no significant effect of carvedilol on outcome.[77]

Table 4.2 Randomized trials of pharmacological intervention in ACHD

Author	Year	Population	Design	Drug	Sample size	Duration of therapy	Result
Dore et al.[72]	2005	TGA post atrial switch and ccTGA	Multicenter, randomized, double-blind, placebo-controlled, crossover	Losartan	29	106 days	No improvement of exercise capacity and no reduction in NT-proBNP levels
Kouatli et al.[73]	1997	Fontan	Randomized	Enalapril	18	10 weeks	No benefit in exercise time, cardiac index, or echo parameters of diastolic function
Lester et al.[74]	2001	TGA post atrial switch	Randomized, controlled, crossover	Losartan	7	8 weeks	Improvement in exercise time, reduction in systemic atrioventricular valve regurgitation
Babu-Narayan et al.[75]	2006	Tetralogy of Fallot and pulmonary regurgitation	Randomized, double-blind, placebo controlled	Ramipril	64	6 months	No benefit in right or left ventricular ejection fraction, degree of pulmonary regurgitation, neurohormones, or exercise capacity

(*continued*)

Table 4.2 (continued)

Author	Year	Population	Design	Drug	Sample size	Duration of therapy	Result
Therrien et al.[76]	2008	TGA post atrial switch	Randomized, double-blind, placebo controlled	Ramipril	17	1 year	No benefit in right ventricular function assessed by MRI
Shaddy et al.[77]	2007	Children and adolescents, dilated cardiomyopathy or CHD	Multicenter, randomized, double-blind, placebo controlled	Carvedilol	161	8 months	No clinical improvement
Norozi et al.[78]	2007	Tetralogy of Fallot	Randomized, double-blind, placebo controlled	Bisoprolol	33	6 months	No benefit in exercise capacity, natriuretic peptides, right and left ventricular size and function
Galie et al., BREATHE-5[79]	2005	Eisenmenger	Multicenter, randomized, double-blind, placebo controlled	Bosentan	54	16 weeks	Decrease in pulmonary vascular resistance, improved six-minute walking distance and functional class

TGA transposition of the great arteries, *ccTGA* congenitally corrected transposition of the great arteries, *CHD* congenital heart disease

A small case series of three patients with Fontan palliation showed that high-dose spironolactone may be helpful in the remission of protein-losing enteropathy.[86]

4.5.3 Targeting Pulmonary Arterial Hypertension

Recently, new therapies have become available for patients with pulmonary arterial hypertension, including those with ACHD. Epoprostenol has been shown to improve functional status, systemic saturations and pulmonary hemodynamics in patients with congenital heart disease and pulmonary arterial hypertension.[87] Epoprostenol is, however, limited by the need for intravenous administration and consequent complications such as line and systemic infections. Bosentan, an oral dual-receptor endothelin antagonist, improved exercise capacity in patients with Eisenmenger syndrome in several open-label intention-to-treat pilot studies and in a recent randomized placebo-controlled study (BREATHE-5).[79] Sildenafil, an oral phospodiasterase-5-inhibitor, improves functional capacity in patients with pulmonary arterial hypertension, including some with congenital heart disease. A small randomized trial of sildenafil in ten Eisenmenger patients found a significant improvement in functional status, exercise capacity and pulmonary pressures in the Eisenmenger subgroup.[88] Oral administration of a single dose of sildenafil acutely improved exercise capacity and hemodynamic response to exercise in 27 patients with Fontan circulation.[89] Other large randomized trials using treprostinil,[90] sildenafil[91] and sitaxsentan[92,93] have included a minority of patients with ACHD in their population. A minority of ACHD patients were also included in the recently published EARLY study assessing the effect of bosentan on patients with pulmonary arterial hypertension in functional class II.[94] None of these studies, however, was powered for formal subgroup analysis, leaving doubts on the applicability of their results to the ACHD population.[95] Moreover, it still remains unclear whether the beneficial effect on these therapies on exercise capacity and clinical status translates into a survival benefit. Finally, it remains unclear whether selected patients in whom advanced pulmonary arterial hypertension therapies convey a significant clinical and hemodynamic benefit could safely undergo partial or complete repair of the underlying cardiac defect in a "treat-and-repair" fashion.[63]

4.5.4 Resynchronization

Ventricular dyssynchrony has been found to significantly affect cardiac function and is a target for therapy in patients with left ventricular dysfunction and intraventricular conduction delay.[96–99] While there is mounting evidence that ventricular dyssynchrony is present in patients with congenital heart disease, randomized trials of resynchronization in this population are lacking.[99–101]

Preliminary studies of ventricular resynchronization in congenital cohorts have been promising. An increase in systolic blood pressure and cardiac index was reported with biventricular pacing during the post-operative period in biventricular hearts with significant intraventricular delay.[102,103] Dubin et al. showed an acute increase in cardiac output and right ventricular systolic performance in patients with intraventricular delay.[104] Registries have reported beneficial clinical effects of resynchronization on functional capacity, as well on systemic ventricular function and QRS duration.[105,106]

Implantation of cardiac resynchronization devices in ACHD patients may present significant difficulties due to the varying intracardiac anatomy and should be performed by appropriately trained operators. The role of resynchronization, like that of implantable cardioverter-defibrillators, in the setting of ACHD needs to be explored further by clinical trials.[107]

4.5.5 Other Therapies

Diuretics are the first line of treatment for signs and symptoms of congestive heart failure, both in congenital and non-congenital heart disease. However, care should be taken to avoid dehydration in ACHD which is often dependent on preload for maintaining right ventricular output and amongst patients with pulmonary arterial hypertension. Anticoagulation or anti-aggregation is also often used in ACHD patients who are deemed at risk of thrombosis and embolic events such as those with severely dilated ventricles, Fontan-type circulation, Eisenmenger syndrome and those with chronic, persistent or recurrent arrhythmias.

Data on supplemental oxygen in patients with cyanotic heart defects are very limited. Oxygen may have a role for nocturnal use in selected patients,[108,109] however, round the clock use in young individuals may lead to "oxygen dependence" causing physical deconditioning and thus, is not advisable. Venesections, performed routinely in cyanotic ACHD patients in the past as a means of reducing the risk of hyperviscosity symptoms and improving functional status, are now thought to be harmful and should be avoided.[110] Rehydration and iron repletion should be the first step towards managing severe hyperviscosity symptoms, which by the way mimic the symptoms of iron deficiency. Interventions such as atrial septectomy, the palliative Mustard operation aimed at reducing cyanosis and improving the functional state of Eisenmenger patients, are rarely used nowadays, but can be effective in appropriately selected patients.

Exercise training has established psychological and physical benefits on patients with acquired heart disease.[55] There are limited data on the effects of exercise training in ACHD, with most available studies concluding that exercise training is safe and may be beneficial.[111,112] The 36th Bethesda conference recommendations for the participation of patients with congenital heart disease in sports suggest the use of exercise testing for assessing the impact of exercise on ACHD patients before advising any level of training in the clinical setting.[113] Simple preventive measures such as avoiding excessive dehydration are also recommended. High-impact sport should be discouraged in patients on anticoagulation therapy or with a pacemaker as well as patients with Marfan's syndrome. Extreme caution is also recommended in patients at high risk of arrhythmia and sudden death such as those with long QT syndrome, arrhythmogenic right ventricular dysplasia and hypertrophic obstructive cardiomyopathy. All recommendations should be thoroughly discussed with patients.

The role of transplantation, heart and/or lung, remains relatively limited in ACHD. The scarcity of donors, the very slow deterioration with a mortality rate significantly lower to that of end-stage acquired heart failure, the high prevalence of complications such as renal and hepatic dysfunction in symptomatic ACHD patients and the often complex cardiovascular anatomy, result in very few patients actually receiving a transplant.[110]

4.6 Future Prospects in ACHD

Evidence-based medicine is the basis of modern practice in cardiology. Both heart failure and ischemic heart disease are now treated following recommendations based on strong clinical evidence deriving, mainly, from randomized controlled trials. Treatment of pediatric and ACHD patients, however, remains largely empirical, as little evidence is available on which to base clinical decisions. Randomized controlled trials are clearly needed in ACHD to rationalize treatment in this population.[4] Most randomized trials in this field have been too small to demonstrate a beneficial effect of therapies, such as trials with ACE-inhibitors. Despite the exponential increase in the number of ACHD patients followed at specialist centers, the absolute number of patients with individual ACHD diagnoses remains low, with significant within-group heterogeneity (different prior interventions, range of anatomy or associated lesions, etc.). Thus, the required sample size for performing studies in ACHD often exceeds the number of available participants in a single center, hence the need for multicenter collaboration.[114,115]

Recruitment of patients and selection of appropriate endpoints may also be problematic in ACHD. Many patients receive empirical treatment reducing the number of potential candidates resulting in the inclusion of patients at the best end of the spectrum, which reduces the chances of observing a rapid, sizable effect of the intervention. Moreover, the rate of "hard" endpoints such as mortality is often low in ACHD and surrogate markers of outcome such as ventricular function or exercise capacity are used, introducing additional noise related to reproducibility of measurements, and cost.[116] Careful selection of endpoints to ensure adequate patient participation and compliance to protocol are thus paramount. Education of patients on the importance of trials and the potential benefits to themselves is equally important.[117,118] Pharmacological therapy in ACHD patients should, whenever possible, occur within prospective protocols, ideally in multicenter studies or registries. Studies with longer follow-up could compensate for the lack of power and low event rates, allowing for the use of "hard" endpoints.

4.7 Conclusions

Chronic heart failure is widely prevalent in congenital heart disease. It is in most cases multifactorial. Although most previous interventions for ACHD have transformed the prospects for these patients, the intervention/s themselves have not been truly curative.

Chronic heart failure in ACHD represents multiple potential therapeutic opportunities, which need to be explored in prospective studies.

Acknowledgments Dr. Dimopoulos has been supported by the European Society of Cardiology. Dr. Giannakoulas was supported from the Hellenic Heart Foundation, the Hellenic Cardiological Society, the Propondis Foundation and the DG Education & Culture- LLP Programme-Leonardo Da Vinci Mobility. Prof Gatzoulis and the Royal Brompton Adult Congenital Heart Programme and the Department of Clinical Cardiology have received support from the British Heart Foundation and the Clinical Research Committee, Royal Brompton Hospital, London, United Kingdom.

References

1. Dickstein K, Cohen-Solal A, Filippatos G et al. ESC Guidelines for the diagnosis and treatment of acute and chronic heart failure 2008: the Task Force for the Diagnosis and Treatment of Acute and Chronic Heart Failure 2008 of the European Society of Cardiology. Developed in collaboration with the Heart Failure Association of the ESC (HFA) and endorsed by the European Society of Intensive Care Medicine (ESICM). *Eur Heart J.* 2008;29:2388–2442.
2. Hunt SA. ACC/AHA 2005 guideline update for the diagnosis and management of chronic heart failure in the adult: a report of the American College of Cardiology/American Heart Association Task Force on Practice Guidelines (Writing Committee to Update the 2001 Guidelines for the Evaluation and Management of Heart Failure). *J Am Coll Cardiol.* 2005;46:e1–e82.
3. Bolger AP, Coats AJ, Gatzoulis MA. Congenital heart disease: the original heart failure syndrome. *Eur Heart J.*2003; 24:970–976.
4. Dimopoulos K, Diller GP, Piepoli MF et al. Exercise intolerance in adults with congenital heart disease. *Cardiol Clin.*2006; 24:641–660,vi i.
5. Engelfriet P, Tijssen J, Kaemmerer H et al. Adherence to guidelines in the clinical care for adults with congenital heart disease: the Euro Heart Survey on adult congenital heart disease. *Eur Heart J.*2006; 27:737–745.
6. Veldtman GR, Nishimoto A, Siu S et al. The Fontan procedure in adults. *Heart.* 2001; 86:330–335.
7. Diller GP, Dimopoulos K, Okonko D et al. Exercise intolerance in adult congenital heart disease: comparative severity, correlates, and prognostic implication. *Circulation.* 2005;112:828–835.
8. Dimopoulos K, Okonko DO, Diller GP et al. Abnormal ventilatory response to exercise in adults with congenital heart disease relates to cyanosis and predicts survival. *Circulation.* 2006;113:2796–2802.
9. Graham TP, Jr., Bernard YD, Mellen BG et al. Long-term outcome in congenitally corrected transposition of the great arteries: a multi-institutional study. *J Am Coll Cardiol.* 2000; 36:255–261.
10. Puley G, Siu S, Connelly M et al. Arrhythmia and survival in patients >18 years of age after the mustard procedure for complete transposition of the great arteries. *Am J Cardiol.* 1999; 83:1080–1084.
11. Piran S, Veldtman G, Siu S et al. Heart failure and ventricular dysfunction in patients with single or systemic right ventricles. *Circulation.*2002; 105:1189–1194.
12. Fredriksen PM, Veldtman G, Hechter S et al. Aerobic capacity in adults with various congenital heart diseases. *Am J Cardiol.*2001; 87:310–314.
13. Bolger AP, Gatzoulis MA. Towards defining heart failure in adults with congenital heart disease. *Int J Cardiol.*2004; 97(suppl1) :15–23.

14. Davlouros PA, Kilner PJ, Hornung TS et al. Right ventricular function in adults with repaired tetralogy of Fallot assessed with cardiovascular magnetic resonance imaging: detrimental role of right ventricular outflow aneurysms or akinesia and adverse right-to-left ventricular interaction. *J Am Coll Cardiol.*2002; 40:2044–2052.
15. Warnes CA, Somerville J. Tricuspid atresia in adolescents and adults: current state and late complications. *Br Heart J.*1986; 56:535–543.
16. Clark AL, Poole-Wilson PA, Coats AJ. Exercise limitation in chronic heart failure: central role of the periphery. *J Am Coll Cardiol.*1996; 28:1092–1102.
17. Giardini A, Specchia S, Berton E et al. Strong and independent prognostic value of peak circulatory power in adults with congenital heart disease. *Am Heart J.*2007; 154:441–447.
18. Wasserman K. *Principles of Exercise Testing and Interpretation Including Pathophysiology and Clinical Applications*. Philadelphia, PA: Lippincott Williams & Wilkins; 2005.
19. ATS/ACCP. Statement on cardiopulmonary exercise testing. 2003;167:211–277.
20. Diller GP, Dimopoulos K, Benson LR et al. Ventilatory efficiency and heart rate response are the strongest exercise markers of outcome in noncyanotic adults with congenital heart disease. J Am Coll Cardiol. 2007;49:A268.
21. Gitt AK, Wasserman K, Kilkowski C et al. Exercise anaerobic threshold and ventilatory efficiency identify heart failure patients for high risk of early death. *Circulation.* 2002;106:3079–3084.
22. Glaser S, Opitz CF, Bauer U et al. Assessment of symptoms and exercise capacity in cyanotic patients with congenital heart disease. *Chest.*2004; 125:368–376.
23. Frigiola A, Tsang V, Bull C et al. Biventricular response after pulmonary valve replacement for right ventricular outflow tract dysfunction: is age a predictor of outcome? *Circulation.* 2008;118:S182–S190.
24. Niedeggen A, Skobel E, Haager P et al. Comparison of the 6-minute walk test with established parameters for assessment of cardiopulmonary capacity in adults with complex congenital cardiac disease. *Cardiol Young.*2005; 15:385–390.
25. Weber KT, Janicki JS, McElroy PA. Determination of aerobic capacity and the severity of chronic cardiac and circulatory failure. *Circulation.*1987; 76:VI40–VI45.
26. Cullen S, Shore D, Redington A. Characterization of right ventricular diastolic performance after complete repair of tetralogy of Fallot. Restrictive physiology predicts slow postoperative recovery. *Circulation.*1995; 91:1782–1789.
27. Zhu Y, Gramolini AO, Walsh MA et al. Tbx5-dependent pathway regulating diastolic function in congenital heart disease. *Proc Natl Acad Sci U S A.*20 08;105:5519–5524.
28. Giannakoulas G, Dimopoulos K, Engel R et al. Burden of coronary artery disease in adults with congenital heart disease and its relation to congenital and traditional heart risk factors. *Am J Cardiol.*2009; 103:1445–1450.
29. Diller GP, Dimopoulos K, Okonko D et al. Heart rate response during exercise predicts survival in adults with congenital heart disease. *J Am Coll Cardiol.*2006; 48:1250–1256.
30. Norozi K, Wessel A, Alpers V et al. Chronotropic incompetence in adolescents and adults with congenital heart disease after cardiac surgery. *J Card Fail.*2007; 13:263–268.
31. Diller GP, Okonko DO, Uebing A et al. Impaired heart rate response to exercise in adult patients with a systemic right ventricle or univentricular circulation: Prevalence, relation to exercise, and potential therapeutic implications. *Int J Cardiol.*2008: 59–66.
32. Kaltman JR, Ro PS, Zimmerman F et al. Managed ventricular pacing in pediatric patients and patients with congenital heart disease. *Am J Cardiol.*200 8;102:875–878.
33. Spence MS, Balaratnam MS, Gatzoulis MA. Clinical update: cyanotic adult congenital heart disease. *Lancet.*2007; 370:1530–1532.
34. Bolger AP, Sharma R, Li W et al. Neurohormonal activation and the chronic heart failure syndrome in adults with congenital heart disease. *Circulation.*2002; 106:92–99.
35. Hopkins WE, Chen Z, Fukagawa NK et al. Increased atrial and brain natriuretic peptides in adults with cyanotic congenital heart disease: enhanced understanding of the relationship between hypoxia and natriuretic peptide secretion. *Circulation.*2004; 109:2872–2877.

36. Davos CH, Davlouros PA, Wensel R et al. Global impairment of cardiac autonomic nervous activity late after repair of tetralogy of Fallot. *Circulation.*2002; 106:I69–175.
37. Davos CH, Francis DP, Leenarts MF et al. Global impairment of cardiac autonomic nervous activity late after the Fontan operation. *Circulation.*2003; 108(suppl1) :II180–II185.
38. Niwa K, Tateno S, Akagi T et al. Arrhythmia and reduced heart rate variability during pregnancy in women with congenital heart disease and previous reparative surgery. *Int J Cardiol.* 2007;122:143–148.
39. Tateno S, Niwa K, Nakazawa M et al. Arrhythmia and conduction disturbances in patients with congenital heart disease during pregnancy: multicenter study. *Circ J.* 2003;67:992–997.
40. Lammers A, Kaemmerer H, Hollweck R et al. Impaired cardiac autonomic nervous activity predicts sudden cardiac death in patients with operated and unoperated congenital cardiac disease. *J Thorac Cardiovasc Surg.*2006; 132:647–655.
41. Mancini DM, Henson D, LaManca J et al. Evidence of reduced respiratory muscle endurance in patients with heart failure. *J Am Coll Cardiol.*1994; 24:972–981.
42. Anker SD, Swan JW, Volterrani M et al. The influence of muscle mass, strength, fatigability and blood flow on exercise capacity in cachectic and non-cachectic patients with chronic heart failure. *Eur Heart J.*1997; 18:259–269.
43. Sullivan MJ, Green HJ, Cobb FR. Skeletal muscle biochemistry and histology in ambulatory patients with long-term heart failure. *Circulation.*1990 ;81:518–527.
44. Massie BM, Conway M, Rajagopalan B et al. Skeletal muscle metabolism during exercise under ischemic conditions in congestive heart failure. Evidence for abnormalities unrelated to blood flow. *Circulation.*1988; 78:320–326.
45. Coats AJ, Clark AL, Piepoli M et al. Symptoms and quality of life in heart failure: the muscle hypothesis. *Br Heart J.*1994; 72:S36–S39.
46. Piepoli M, Clark AL, Volterrani M et al. Contribution of muscle afferents to the hemodynamic, autonomic, and ventilatory responses to exercise in patients with chronic heart failure: effects of physical training. *Circulation.*1996; 93:940–952.
47. Coats AJS. Origin of symptoms in patients with cachexia with special reference to weakness and shortness of breath. *Int J Cardiol.*2002; 85:133–139.
48. Scott AC, Davies LC, Coats AJ et al. Relationship of skeletal muscle metaboreceptors in the upper and lower limbs with the respiratory control in patients with heart failure. *Clin Sci (Lond).*2002;102: 23–30.
49. Brassard P, Poirier P, Martin J et al. Impact of exercise training on muscle function and ergoreflex in Fontan patients: a pilot study. *Int J Cardiol.*2006; 107:85–94.
50. Georgiadou P, Babu-Narayan SV, Francis DP et al. Periodic breathing as a feature of right heart failure in congenital heart disease. *Heart.*2004; 90:1075–1076.
51. Vonder Muhll IF, Cholet A, Stehr K et al. Increased metabolic rate as a mechanism for cachexia in adults with congenital heart disease. *J Am Coll Cardiol.*2004; 43(supplA):384.
52. Hambrecht R, Niebauer J, Fiehn E et al. Physical training in patients with stable chronic heart failure: effects on cardiorespiratory fitness and ultrastructural abnormalities of leg muscles. *J Am Coll Cardiol.*1995; 25:1239–1249.
53. Adamopoulos S, Coats AJ, Brunotte F et al. Physical training improves skeletal muscle metabolism in patients with chronic heart failure. *J Am Coll Cardiol.*1993; 21:1101–1106.
54. Sullivan MJ, Higginbotham MB, Cobb FR. Exercise training in patients with chronic heart failure delays ventilatory anaerobic threshold and improves submaximal exercise performance. *Circulation.*1989; 79:324–329.
55. Piepoli MF, Davos C, Francis DP et al. Exercise training meta-analysis of trials in patients with chronic heart failure (ExTraMATCH). *BMJ.*2004 ;328:189.
56. Clark A, Coats A. The mechanisms underlying the increased ventilatory response to exercise in chronic stable heart failure. *Eur Heart J.*1992; 13:1698–1708.
57. Francis DP, Shamim W, Davies LC et al. Cardiopulmonary exercise testing for prognosis in chronic heart failure: continuous and independent prognostic value from VE/VCO(2)slope and peak VO(2). *Eur Heart J.*2000; 21:154–161.

58. Sharma R, Bolger AP, Li W et al. Elevated circulating levels of inflammatory cytokines and bacterial endotoxin in adults with congenital heart disease. *Am J Cardiol.* 2003;92: 188–193.
59. Oechslin E, Kiowski W, Schindler R et al. Systemic endothelial dysfunction in adults with cyanotic congenital heart disease. *Circulation.*2005; 112:1106–1112.
60. Diller GP, van Eijl S, Okonko DO et al. Circulating endothelial progenitor cells in patients with Eisenmenger syndrome and idiopathic pulmonary arterial hypertension. *Circulation.* 2008;117:3020–3030.
61. Dimopoulos K, Diller GP, Koltsida E et al. Prevalence, predictors, and prognostic value of renal dysfunction in adults with congenital heart disease. *Circulation.*2008; 117:2320–2328.
62. Dimopoulos K, Diller JP, Petraco R et al. Hyponatremia in adults with congenital heart disease: prevalence and relation to outcome. *Eur Heart J.*2008; 29(suppl):744.
63. Dimopoulos K, Peset A, Gatzoulis MA. Evaluating operability in adults with congenital heart disease and the role of pretreatment with targeted pulmonary arterial hypertension therapy. *Int J Cardiol.*2008;12 9:163–171.
64. Mott AR, Feltes TF, McKenzie ED et al. Improved early results with the Fontan operation in adults with functional single ventricle. *Ann Thorac Surg.*2004; 77:1334–1340.
65. Borowski A, Ghodsizad A, Litmathe J et al. Severe pulmonary regurgitation late after total repair of tetralogy of Fallot: surgical considerations. *Pediatr Cardiol.*2004; 25:466–471.
66. Brown JW, Ruzmetov M, Vijay P et al. Surgical repair of congenital supravalvular aortic stenosis in children. *Eur J Cardiothorac Surg.*2002; 21:50–56.
67. Masetti P, Ussia GP, Gazzolo D et al. Aortic pulmonary autograft implant: medium-term follow-up with a note on a new right ventricular pulmonary artery conduit. *J Card Surg.* 1998;13:173–176.
68. Brochu MC, Baril JF, Dore A et al. Improvement in exercise capacity in asymptomatic and mildly symptomatic adults after atrial septal defect percutaneous closure. *Circulation.* 2002;106:1821–1826.
69. Papadopoulou SA, Dimopoulos K, Gatzoulis MA. Near miss sudden cardiac death on a young patient with repaired atrioventricular septal defect. *Int J Cardiol.*2008; 130:e117–118.
70. Shaddy RE, Webb G. Applying heart failure guidelines to adult congenital heart disease patients. *Expert Rev Cardiovasc Ther.*2008; 6:165–174.
71. Dimopoulos K. Trials and tribulations in adult congenital heart disease. *Int J Cardiol.* 2008;129:160–162.
72. Dore A, Houde C, Chan KL et al. Angiotensin receptor blockade and exercise capacity in adults with systemic right ventricles: a multicenter, randomized, placebo-controlled clinical trial. *Circulation.*2 005;112:2411–2416.
73. Kouatli AA, Garcia JA, Zellers TM et al. Enalapril does not enhance exercise capacity in patients after Fontan procedure. *Circulation.*1997; 96:1507–1512.
74. Lester SJ, McElhinney DB, Viloria E et al. Effects of losartan in patients with a systemically functioning morphologic right ventricle after atrial repair of transposition of the great arteries. *Am J Cardiol.*2001; 88:1314–1316.
75. Babu-Narayan SV, Uebing A, Davlouros PA et al. ACE inhibitors for potential prevention of the deleterious effects of pulmonary regurgitation in adults with tetralogy of Fallot repair – the appropriate study - a randomised double-blinded placebo-controlled trial in adults with congenital heart disease. *Circulation.*2006; 114(suppll I):409.
76. Therrien J, Provost Y, Harrison J et al. Effect of angiotensin receptor blockade on systemic right ventricular function and size: a small, randomized, placebo-controlled study. *Int J Cardiol.*2008;129: 187–192.
77. Shaddy RE, Boucek MM, Hsu DT et al. Carvedilol for children and adolescents with heart failure: a randomized controlled trial. *JAMA.*2007; 298:1171–1179.
78. Norozi K, Bahlmann J, Raab B et al. A prospective, randomized, double-blind, placebo controlled trial of beta-blockade in patients who have undergone surgical correction of tetralogy of Fallot. *Cardiol Young.*2007; 17:372–379.

79. Galie N, Beghetti M, Gatzoulis MA et al. Bosentan therapy in patients with Eisenmenger syndrome: a multicenter, double-blind, randomized, placebo-controlled study. *Circulation*. 2006;114:48–54.
80. Heragu N, Mahony L. Is captopril useful in decreasing pleural drainage in children after modified Fontan operation? *Am J Cardiol*.1999; 84:1109–1112,A 1110.
81. Hechter SJ, Fredriksen PM, Liu P et al. Angiotensin-converting enzyme inhibitors in adults after the Mustard procedure. *Am J Cardiol*.2001; 87:660–663,A 611.
82. Hopkins WE, Kelly DP. Angiotensin-converting enzyme inhibitors in adults with cyanotic congenital heart disease. *Am J Cardiol*.1996; 77:439–440.
83. Buchhorn R, Bartmus D, Siekmeyer W et al. Beta-blocker therapy of severe congestive heart failure in infants with left to right shunts. *Am J Cardiol*.1998; 81:1366–1368.
84. Matsuyama K, Ueda Y, Ogino H et al. beta-blocker therapy in patients after aortic valve replacement for aortic regurgitation. *Int J Cardiol*.200 0;73:49–53.
85. Giardini A, Lovato L, Donti A et al. A pilot study on the effects of carvedilol on right ventricular remodelling and exercise tolerance in patients with systemic right ventricle. *Int J Cardiol*. 2006.
86. Ringel RE, Peddy SB. Effect of high-dose spironolactone on protein-losing enteropathy in patients with Fontan palliation of complex congenital heart disease. *Am J Cardiol*. 2003;91: 1031–1032,A 1039.
87. Rosenzweig EB, Kerstein D, Barst RJ. Long-term prostacyclin for pulmonary hypertension with associated congenital heart defects. *Circulation*.1999; 99:1858–1865.
88. Singh TP, Rohit M, Grover A et al. A randomized, placebo-controlled, double-blind, crossover study to evaluate the efficacy of oral sildenafil therapy in severe pulmonary artery hypertension. *Am Heart J*.2006; 151:851e 851–e855.
89. Giardini A, Balducci A, Specchia S et al. Effect of sildenafil on haemodynamic response to exercise and exercise capacity in Fontan patients. *Eur Heart J*.2008; 29:1681–1687.
90. Simonneau G, Barst RJ, Galie N et al. Continuous subcutaneous infusion of treprostinil, a prostacyclin analogue, in patients with pulmonary arterial hypertension: a double-blind, randomized, placebo-controlled trial. *Am J Respir Crit Care Med*.2002; 165:800–804.
91. Galie N, Ghofrani HA, Torbicki A et al. Sildenafil citrate therapy for pulmonary arterial hypertension. *N Engl J Med*.2005; 353:2148–2157.
92. Barst RJ, Langleben D, Badesch D et al. Treatment of pulmonary arterial hypertension with the selective endothelin-A receptor antagonist sitaxsentan. *J Am Coll Cardiol*. 2006;47: 2049–2056.
93. Barst RJ, Langleben D, Frost A et al. Sitaxsentan therapy for pulmonary arterial hypertension. *Am J Respir Crit Care Med*.2004; 169:441–447.
94. Galie N, Rubin L, Hoeper M et al. Treatment of patients with mildly symptomatic pulmonary arterial hypertension with bosentan (EARLY study): a double-blind, randomised controlled trial. *Lancet*.200 8;371:2093–2100.
95. Giannakoulas G, Dimopoulos K, Gatzoulis MA. Bosentan in mild pulmonary hypertension. *Lancet*. 2008;372:1730–1731; author reply 1731.
96. Bristow MR, Saxon LA, Boehmer J et al. Cardiac-resynchronization therapy with or without an implantable defibrillator in advanced chronic heart failure. *N Engl J Med*. 2004; 350:2140–2150.
97. Young JB, Abraham WT, Smith AL et al. Combined cardiac resynchronization and implantable cardioversion defibrillation in advanced chronic heart failure: the MIRACLE ICD Trial. *JAMA*.2003;289 :2685–2694.
98. Cazeau S, Leclercq C, Lavergne T et al. Effects of multisite biventricular pacing in patients with heart failure and intraventricular conduction delay. *N Engl J Med*.2001; 344:873–880.
99. Uebing A, Gibson DG, Babu-Narayan SV et al. Right ventricular mechanics and QRS duration in patients with repaired tetralogy of Fallot: implications of infundibular disease. *Circulation*.2007; 116:1532–1539.

100. Friedberg MK, Silverman NH, Dubin AM et al. Right ventricular mechanical dyssynchrony in children with hypoplastic left heart syndrome. *J Am Soc Echocardiogr.* 2007;20: 1073–1079.
101. Chow PC, Liang XC, Lam WW et al.Mechanical right ventricular dyssynchrony in patients after atrial switch operation for transposition of the great arteries. *Am J Cardiol.* 2008;101:874–881.
102. Janousek J, Vojtovic P, Hucin B et al. Resynchronization pacing is a useful adjunct to the management of acute heart failure after surgery for congenital heart defects. *Am J Cardiol.* 2001;88:145–152.
103. Zimmerman FJ, Starr JP, Koenig PR et al. Acute hemodynamic benefit of multisite ventricular pacing after congenital heart surgery. *Ann Thorac Surg.* 2003;75:1775–1780.
104. Dubin AM, Feinstein JA, Reddy VM et al. Electrical resynchronization: a novel therapy for the failing right ventricle. *Circulation.* 2003;107:2287–2289.
105. Dubin AM, Janousek J, Rhee E et al. Resynchronization therapy in pediatric and congenital heart disease patients: an international multicenter study. *J Am Coll Cardiol.* 2005;46: 2277–2283.
106. Cecchin F, Frangini PA, Brown DW et al. Cardiac resynchronization therapy (and multisite pacing) in pediatrics and congenital heart disease: five years experience in a single institution. *J Cardiovasc Electrophysiol.* 2009;20:58–65.
107. Saul JP, Epstein AE, Silka MJ et al. Heart Rhythm Society/Pediatric and Congenital Electrophysiology Society Clinical Competency Statement: training pathways for implantation of cardioverter-defibrillators and cardiac resynchronization therapy devices in pediatric and congenital heart patients. *Heart Rhythm.* 2008;5:926–933.
108. Bowyer JJ, Busst CM, Denison DM et al. Effect of long term oxygen treatment at home in children with pulmonary vascular disease. *Br Heart J.* 1986;55:385–390.
109. Sandoval J, Aguirre JS, Pulido T et al. Nocturnal oxygen therapy in patients with the Eisenmenger syndrome. *Am J Respir Crit Care Med.* 2001;164:1682–1687.
110. Dimopoulos K, Giannakoulas G, Wort SJ et al. Pulmonary arterial hypertension in adults with congenital heart disease: distinct differences from other causes of pulmonary arterial hypertension and management implications. *Curr Opin Cardiol.* 2008;23:545–554.
111. Thaulow E, Fredriksen PM. Exercise and training in adults with congenital heart disease. *Int J Cardiol.* 2004;97(suppl 1):35–38.
112. Therrien J, Fredriksen P, Walker M et al. A pilot study of exercise training in adult patients with repaired tetralogy of Fallot. *Can J Cardiol.* 2003;19:685–689.
114. Schulz KF, Grimes DA. Sample size calculations in randomised trials: mandatory and mystical. *Lancet.* 2005;365:1348–1353.
113. Graham TP, Jr., Driscoll DJ, Gersony WM et al. Task Force 2: congenital heart disease. *J Am Coll Cardiol.* 2005;45:1326–1333.
115. Gatzoulis MA, Webb GD, Daubeney PEF. *Diagnosis and Management of Adult Congenital Heart Disease.* Edinburgh: Churchill Livingstone; 2003.
116. Konstam MA, Udelson JE, Anand IS et al. Ventricular remodeling in heart failure: a credible surrogate endpoint. *J Card Fail.* 2003;9:350–353.
117. Gatzoulis MA. Adult congenital heart disease: education, education, education. *Nat Clin Pract Cardiovasc Med.* 2006;3:2–3.
118. Caldwell PH, Murphy SB, Butow PN et al. Clinical trials in children. *Lancet.* 2004;364:803–811.

5 Indications and Outcomes of Heart Transplantation in the Patient with Congenital Heart Disease

Charles E. Canter

The year 2008 marks the fortieth anniversary of the utilization of heart transplantation as therapy for congenital heart disease.[1] Since the introduction of cyclosporine-based immunosuppression over 20 years ago,[2,3] heart transplantation has evolved from a heroic therapy to a widely applied therapy for patients with congenital heart disease from infancy to adulthood. Within the International Society for Heart and Lung Transplantation (ISHLT) database, patients with congenital heart disease account for 50–75% of the transplants performed in infants <1 year of age; 25–50% of the transplants performed in children 1–10 years of age; and approximately 25% of the transplants performed in adolescents 10–17 years of age (Fig. 5.1).[4] Patients with congenital heart disease account for only 3% of adult (>18 years of age) heart transplants in the ISHLT database.[5]

Heart transplantation is utilized in congenital heart disease as both primary therapy and as "rescue" therapy for end-stage heart failure after previous surgical reparative or palliative procedures. Heart transplantation as primary therapy almost exclusively occurs in infancy, but continues to be performed rarely even in adults.[6] Heart transplantation as rescue therapy may occur both for intractable heart failure after an acutely unsuccessful surgical repair or palliation, and also for end-stage heart failure occurring months to years (even decades) after initially successful surgical procedures. This chapter will explore transplantation in patients with congenital heart disease as it relates to (1) the clinical scenarios where heart transplantation is currently thought to be useful and indicated; (2) outcomes during the waiting period prior to transplant, and (3) outcomes after transplantation has occurred.

5.1 Indications for Heart Transplantation as Primary Therapy for Congenital Heart Disease

Improvements in immunosuppression with the introduction of cyclosporine, animal research suggesting a decreased immunologic response to heart transplantation in infants, and the poor results with palliative surgery for hypoplastic left heart syndrome led

C.E. Canter
Professor of Pediatrics, Washington University School of Medicine, Medical Director, Heart Failure and Transplant Program, St. Louis Children's Hospital

R.E. Shaddy (ed.), *Heart Failure in Congenital Heart Disease*,
DOI: 10.1007/978-1-84996-480-7_5, © Springer-Verlag London Limited 2011

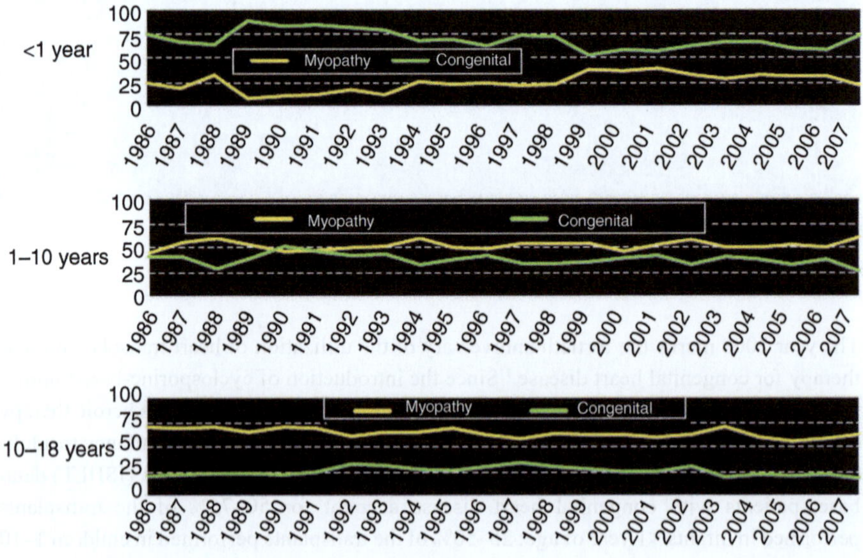

Fig. 5.1 Proportions of infants, children, and adolescents undergoing heart transplantation for cardiomyopathy and congenital heart disease from 1986–2007[4]

Leonard Bailey to apply heart transplantation as primary therapy for hypoplastic left heart syndrome in the 1980s.[7] His initial success was rapidly replicated in other centers.[8–10] Many of his initial hypotheses about an immunologic "window of opportunity" for transplantation in infancy have been partially confirmed by clinical experience in the last two decades, demonstrating that infant heart transplant recipients are at a decreased risk for rejection[11,12] and transplant coronary artery disease.[13,14] Infant heart transplant recipients demonstrate the best graft survival rates of any age group in the ISHLT database.[4,5] These outcomes led early consensus conferences[15,16] to list "complex congenital heart disease unamenable to conventional surgical repair or palliation or where the surgical procedure carried a higher risk of mortality than transplantation" as an accepted indication for heart transplantation in pediatric patients.

Outcomes with primary transplantation continued to compare favorably with the results of staged, palliative surgery for hypoplastic left heart syndrome through the 1990s.[17,18] Application of decision analysis modeling in this era,[19] however, suggested the survival advantage of primary transplantation over staged, palliative surgery for hypoplastic left heart syndrome was dependent on both the mortality of staged, palliative procedures *and* the availability of donor organs, which in the United States has been relatively fixed.[20] Thus as the outcomes with staged, palliative surgery have continued to improve,[21–23] primary transplantation for hypoplastic left heart syndrome has declined.[24] An increasing number of infant heart transplants are being performed in patients with cardiomyopathies (Fig. 5.1)[4]; and recent consensus statements on indications for pediatric heart transplantation no longer support transplantation as routine primary therapy for hypoplastic left heart syndrome or any other specific congenital heart lesion.[25]

While the use of heart transplantation as primary therapy for hypoplastic left heart syndrome is declining, certain specific factors related to an individual's congenital heart defect(s) may so significantly increase the risk of death with palliative surgery as to continue to make primary heart transplantation an attractive option. The complex constellation of congenital heart lesions seen with heterotaxy lesions continue to make them high risk candidates for palliative surgery, especially when severe neonatal valve abnormalities are present.[26] This may lead to primary transplantation having a survival advantage over palliative surgery in some cases.[27] Some severe variants of Ebstein's anomaly[28] may also be better served with primary transplantation. In pulmonary atresia with intact ventricular septum, coronary anomalies frequently occur[29] and the coronary circulation may be dependent on the right ventricle. These patients are at higher risk for early death even with successful palliative surgery and have, in some instances, remained candidates for primary transplantation.[30–32] Primary transplantation continues to be recommended as the procedure of choice by some authors[29,30] for infants born with pulmonary atresia with intact ventricular septum and associated coronary ostial atresia.

In rare patients with hypoplastic left heart syndrome, a severely dysmorphic pulmonary valve has complicated successful palliation and led to a decision to proceed with primary transplantation. Hypoplastic left heart syndrome associated with aortic atresia/mitral stenosis has continued to be associated with a higher mortality with staged palliative surgery.[33] A recent study[34] identified the presence of left ventricle-subepicardial coronary artery communications in approximately 50% of this anatomic subtype. Survival with palliative surgery in these patients was only 50% compared to a 94% survival without coronary fistulae, suggesting primary transplantation may remain a viable option for this particular variant of hypoplastic left heart syndrome.

5.2 Indications for Heart Transplantation in Previously Palliated or Repaired Congenital Heart Disease

Most patients who were born with congenital heart disease and undergo heart transplantation do so after some attempt at surgical palliation and/or repair. The Pediatric Heart Transplant Study (PHTS) and Cardiac Transplant Research Database (CTRD) together demonstrated that only 7% of patients older than 6 months of age with congenital heart disease underwent heart transplantation as their initial surgery.[35] Most of these transplants occur between 6 months to 6 years of age with a secondary peak in adolescence. The CTRD demonstrates that adult heart transplantation associated with congenital heart disease occurs primarily between 20 and 40 years of age.

Table 5.1 demonstrates the distribution of specific congenital heart disease diagnoses from 6 months of age through adulthood in the combined databases. Single ventricle lesions are by far the most common lesion, comprising 36% of the total patient group. Heart transplantation may occur at any stage of surgical palliation in these lesions from initial operation, through the cavopulmonary anastomosis, and years after completion of the Fontan procedure.[24,35–39] A morphologic right ventricle serving as a systemic ventricle

Table 5.1 Distribution of the types of congenital heart lesions in children greater than 6 months of age and adults undergoing heart transplantation within the PHTS and CTRD databases[6,35]

Diagnosis	n	% of 488
Single ventricle	176	36
D-transposition of the great arteries	58	12
Right ventricular outflow tract lesions	49	10
Ventricular/atrial septal defect	38	8
Left ventricular outflow tract lesions	38	8
L-transposition of the great arteries	39	8
Complete atrioventricular septal defect	37	8
Other	53	11
Total	488	100

has been shown to be associated with a higher risk for heart failure in single ventricle lesions.[40] The risk of heart failure with a morphologic right systemic ventricle is also underscored by its natural history in transposition of the great vessels, regardless of D- or L-looping, which accounts for the highest proportion of 2-ventricle congenital heart lesions in heart transplant recipients.[35] Right ventricular outflow lesions, including tetralogy of Fallot, left ventricular outflow lesions, and various ventricular and/or atrial septal defects comprise most of the other cases.

Heart transplantation becomes the final therapeutic option for patients with congenital heart disease and intractable heart failure due to various combinations of ventricular dysfunction, residual defects, and acquired defects. It is becoming increasingly apparent that long-term (>5 years) survivors of single ventricle surgical palliation have progressive cardiac deterioration leading to heart failure and death (Fig. 5.2).[40,41] Clinical manifestations

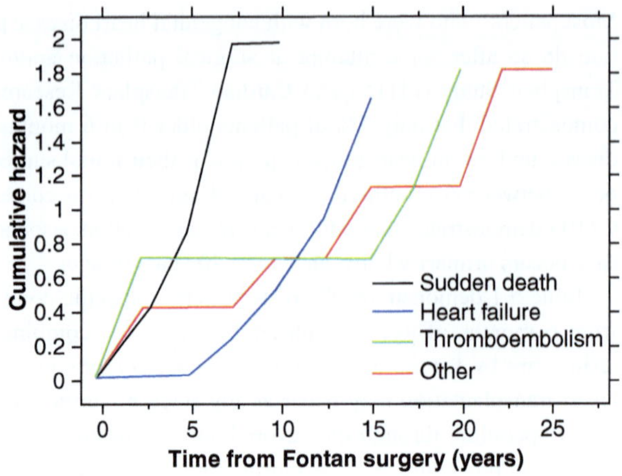

Fig.5. 2 Cumulativeh azard for various causes of death after the Fontan procedure performed at Children's HospitalB oston.[40]H eart failure becomes an important cause of death beginning in patients who survive the first 5y earsa ftert heope ration

of heart failure leading to transplantation range from postoperative cardiogenic shock to "classic" symptoms of dyspnea and reduce exercise tolerance, to more subtle findings of anorexia, nausea, weight loss, and growth failure. While most patients likely have some intrinsic systolic or diastolic myocardial dysfunction, concomitant cardiac morbidities may lead to the presence of intractable heart failure even with minimal to mild ventricular dysfunction. Severe systemic atrioventricular valve insufficiency[42–44] and brady- and/or tachy arrhythmias[42,45–47] are known to increase the risk for progressive heart failure and sudden death in these patients. Persistent cyanosis is highly correlated with poor exercise performance in patients with congenital heart disease.[48] The development of protein-losing enteropathy, which may occur even with relatively low central venous pressures and normal cardiac output in patients after the Fontan procedure, may be debilitating[49,50] and increase the risk for heart failure and death.[40]

Severe heart failure can progress to the point of requiring mechanical circulatory support, mechanical ventilation, and/or intravenous inotropes for effective treatment. This type of severe heart failure has been recognized as a clear cut indication for heart transplantation.[25] However, it becomes much more difficult to determine when heart transplantation is indicated in patients with congenital heart disease whose heart failure does not require such therapies. In pediatric patients, the following are consensus indications for heart transplantation in patients with congenital heart disease: growth failure attributable to heart failure from cardiac disease; intractable arrhythmias unresponsive to treatment with medications, ablation, and/or implantable defibrillators; and a risk for the development of severe irreversible pulmonary vascular disease.[25] Furthermore, the apparent success in the resolution of protein losing enteropathy in Fontan patients after heart transplantation,[38] has increased the enthusiasm for the use of heart transplantation for this complication.[25]

An oxygen consumption treadmill exercise test has been the foundation for determining the indications for heart transplantation in adults with ambulatory heart failure. In "traditional" adult patients with heart failure, a peak oxygen consumption (VO2 max) < 12 cc/kg/min has been associated with a poor 1 year survival rate and a VO2 max > 14 cc/kg/min has a survival rate likely to equal or exceed the survival expected after heart transplantation.[51,52] As the absolute VO2 max can be affected by many factors including age, gender, and body surface area, outcomes in adult patients with heart failure who have <50% predicted VO2 max adjusted for age and sex have been found to correlate with studies using an absolute VO2 max cut point of 14 cc/kg/min.[53–55] For these reasons, adult guidelines[16,56] have generally used either a peak VO2 max < 15 cc/kg/min or < 55% predicted for age and sex as a threshold for candidacy for heart transplantation. Other exercise markers such as enhanced ventilatory response to exercise[57] may also have prognostic value. However, exercise VO2 max level may also reflect skeletal muscle deconditioning.[58] Augmentation of exercise information with other routinely obtained measures affecting outcome in adult patients with heart failure has been used to develop adult heart failure severity scores[59,60] to provide a more accurate assessment of the potential benefits of heart transplantation for an individual patient.

Use of exercise testing for prognostication of outcome in patients with congenital heart disease is challenging in part due to the multiple protocols and instrumentation utilized.[61,62] Measurements of normative VO2 max data in pediatric patients have found that minimum values in patients without heart disease are approximately 60% of predicted values for age and sex.[61] Both patients after Mustard atrial switch repairs of transposition of the great vessels[63] and after the Fontan operation[64] have been shown to have a progressive decrease in exercise tolerance and VO2 max with age. The recently reported results of the Pediatric Heart Network Fontan cohort study showed an average VO2 max of 65% predicted across the group.[65] A patient with congenital heart disease has a perception of physical disability that is frequently much less than what would be anticipated from their measured exercise performance.[66–68] These discrepancies have been attributed to a chronic life-long state of relative cardiac dysfunction. However, recent studies from the Pediatric Heart Network Fontan cohort[65] also demonstrate that submaximal exercise performance is better preserved than maximal performance which could also influence patients' perceptions of disability. This study also found that exercise performance after the Fontan procedure correlated poorly with echocardiographic indices of ventricular function. In aggregate, these findings would suggest that measuring parameters of exercise performance may have limited utility in risk stratification for the determination of the need for heart transplantation in patients with heart failure after previous surgery for congenital heart disease.

A series of studies[48,69,70] from a group investigating adult patients with congenital heart disease in the United Kingdom have suggested that exercise performance may have prognostic value. In their studies[48] VO2 max as a continuous variable was a significant predictor of hospitalization or death, and of death alone. A VO2 max < 15.5 cc/kg/min conferred a higher risk of death (hazard ratio 5.6, 95% CI 1.4–31, $p=0.02$) than higher values. However, the average age of these patients was 33 years compared to the standard older adult patients with heart failure from whom the absolute VO2 max cut point of 14 cc/kg/min was derived. An impaired ventilatory response to exercise (VE/VCO2 slope) was the most powerful predictor of mortality in patients with acyanotic congenital heart disease, but was not useful in cyanotic patients.[69] Finally, a lower heart rate reserve (difference between peak and resting heart rate) predicted mortality independent of antiarrhythmic therapy, functional class, and VO2 max. A lower heart rate reserve was also associated with a significantly greater risk ($p < 0.05$) in patients with complex anatomy, Fontan circulation, and tetralogy of Fallot.[70] Furthermore, it was found that patients with the lowest quartile of heart rate reserve (<51 beats/min) and VO2max (<16.7 cc/kg/min) had the worst prognosis. These findings, if confirmed, suggest that exercise parameters may be of some use as indicators of severity of heart failure in adult patients with congenital heart disease.

5.3 Comorbidities That May Influence Feasibility and Outcomes of Heart Transplantation

The diversity of anomalies of cardiac situs, cardiac position, systemic venous return, pulmonary venous return, pulmonary arteries, and the aorta and its thoracic branches can make heart transplantation in patients with congenital heart disease a daunting technical challenge. These anomalies often require the special expertise of a cardiothoracic surgeon who routinely performs congenital heart surgery. In experienced hands, the special considerations for heart transplantation in virtually all varieties of complex congenital heart disease can be overcome.[71] Thus heart transplantation in patients with congenital heart disease is very rarely unfeasible on technical grounds alone. However, care should be taken for a complete anatomic assessment of cardiac connections prior to transplantation. This assessment may include angiography, vascular ultrasound, magnetic resonance imaging and/or computerized tomography. The goals of this assessment are not only to plan for the surgical procedure, but also to assess vascular access to the heart for the requisite invasive surveillance procedures needed for post-transplant care. Extremely limited venous and/or arterial access to an allograft, which may easily occur in a child after multiple surgical procedures or a prolonged stay in an intensive care unit, may make the needed long-term allograft care and monitoring extremely difficult and be a relative contraindication to transplantation.

The "traditional" comorbidities felt to preclude heart transplantation include irreversible pulmonary, renal, hepatic, or systemic disease; co-existing neoplasm; insulin-dependent diabetes mellitus with end-organ damage; active peptic ulcer disease; and diverticulosis.[15,16,72] Pre-existing renal failure requiring dialysis is a known risk factor for death in pediatric and adult heart transplantation.[4,5] In critically ill pediatric patients on ECMO[73,74] renal failure markedly increases the risk for death after transplantation. Severe pre-existing liver disease can also exist in heart transplant candidates with failed Fontan procedures,[75] and every attempt should be made to distinguish reversible from irreversible cardiac cirrhosis in this patient group. While renal failure and irreversible liver cirrhosis can be contraindications to isolated heart transplantation, initial reports of combined heart-kidney[76,77] or heart-liver[78] transplants are encouraging and may be a viable transplant strategy in these situations.

Cardiac donor allografts are derived from hemodynamic conditions associated with a normally low pulmonary artery pressure and vascular resistance. Placing a relatively deconditioned right ventricle into a pulmonary circuit with high vascular resistance can lead to early postoperative primary graft failure and death.[79–83] Heart transplant candidates with congenital heart disease may have increased pulmonary artery pressure and vascular resistance from a number of mechanisms which may occur in isolation or together, including: left atrial hypertension from systemic ventricular dysfunction and/or atrioventricular valve stenosis or regurgitation; obstruction to pulmonary venous return; pulmonary veno-occlusive disease; pulmonary arteriolar vasoconstriction; obstruction and/or discontinuity of large pulmonary arteries; pulmonary arteriovenous fistulae; intracardiac left-to-right shunts; and extracardiac sources of pulmonary blood flow from a ductus arteriosus or aorto pulmonary collaterals.

While patients with congenital heart disease frequently have elevated pulmonary artery pressure and resistance, experience in these patients[79,84–87] has suggested that such elevations are frequently reversible with a number of medical interventions including prolonged inotropic support and/or pulmonary vasodilators. Furthermore, preliminary experience with pediatric ventricular assist devices (VADs)[88] suggests that such support may lower pulmonary vascular resistance that was not responsive to medical therapy. Current consensus guidelines[25] support the use of heart transplantation in candidates with congenital heart disease and elevated pulmonary vascular resistance if the pulmonary vascular resistance can be lowered to less than 6 Woods units and/or the transpulmonary pressure gradient is less than 15 mm Hg.

The pulmonary circulation in patients with congenital heart disease may have enough multiple anatomic and physiologic complexities to make an accurate measurement of overall pulmonary vascular resistance impossible. Nevertheless, a comprehensive evaluation of the pulmonary circulation is a critical component of the determination of the feasibility of heart transplantation in a patient with congenital heart disease with end-stage heart failure. Heart transplantation has been successfully performed in patients with congenital heart disease where only one lung had a normal pulmonary vascular resistance.[89] Pulmonary arteriovenous fistulae may regress or disappear after transplantation.[90] Careful assessment and (if at all possible) embolization/ligation of aortopulmonary collaterals prior to transplantation may reduce ventricular volume overload and improve cardiac function and symptoms prior to transplantation,[91] in addition to decreasing the risk of primary graft failure due volume overload of the allograft after transplantation.[92]

Pulmonary vascular disease that leads to high levels of fixed pulmonary vascular resistance remains a contraindication to orthotopic heart transplantation,[25] but such patients may be considered for heterotopic heart transplantation[85,93] or heart-lung transplantation. The risk of severe postoperative bleeding associated with the presence of multiple thoracotomies may make heart-lung transplantation problematic. Consideration should also be given for the potential to develop progressive pulmonary vascular disease after transplantation. Patients with heterotaxies and obstructed anomalous pulmonary venous return are at risk for developing progressive pulmonary veno-occlusive disease even after an initial "successful" repair or absence of obstruction in infancy.[94] Fatal pulmonary veno-occlusive disease has also been observed in patients with hypoplastic left heart syndrome born with an intact atrial septum[95] and has led to death even after heart transplantation in infancy.[9]

5.4 Outcomes of Heart Transplant Candidates with Congenital Heart Disease Awaiting Transplantation

The transplant "process" for a patient with congenital heart disease begins when the patient is listed for transplant. "Time zero" for survival is thus most properly measured not from the time of transplantation but from the time of listing. Given the clinical circumstances, it is not surprising that a substantial mortality accrues in heart transplant candidates prior to transplantation. Perhaps the major limitation of heart transplantation as a therapy for end-stage heart failure is the extremely limited supply of donor organs. In the United States,[96] the number of children listed for heart transplantation increases about 1% per year, while the supply of pediatric organ donors has remained static.

Within the PHTS database[97] 14% of the patients listed for transplantation die within 6 months of listing. However, a number of characteristics in the patients listed for heart transplantation affect their risk of death prior to transplant (Fig. 5.4). Increasing severity of heart failure, not unexpectedly, increases the risk of death prior to transplant. Organ allocation algorithms give priority to the sickest patients. In the United States there are three levels of urgency, Status 1A, 1B, and 2, defined by the magnitude of patient support.[98] Currently in the PHTS[97] the 6 month mortality without heart transplantation for candidates listed initially as a Status 1A is 16% and is significantly worse (Fig. 3d) than the 7% 6 month mortality for candidates initially listed as Status 1B and 2% mortality for candidates listed as Status 2. These data can be deceiving, as 50% of patients within the PHTS deteriorate after listing, and die or are transplanted as a Status 1.[99]

Within the group of Status 1A patients, the magnitude of support the candidate requires clearly correlates with mortality while awaiting transplantation. Almond et al.[100] recently analyzed mortality among Status 1A pediatric heart transplant candidates from January 1999 to June 2006 within the American Scientific Registry of Transplant Recipients (SRTR) which is a larger database than the PHTS and encompasses all pediatric transplants in the United States. In the SRTR database, 51% of pediatric Status 1A heart transplant candidates were on inotropic support, 25.4% were on mechanical ventilatory support, and 18% were on extracorporeal membrane oxygenator (ECMO) support at time of listing. While the overall mortality prior to transplant for the group was 21%, the mortality for Status 1A patients only on inotropic support was 14.7%; the mortality for patients initially listed on mechanical ventilation was 25.4%, and the mortality for patients initially listed on ECMO was 31.5%.

Age at listing is also a risk factor for death while awaiting heart transplantation. In both the PHTS (Fig. 5.3a) and the SRTR databases[96] younger children listed for heart transplantation, especially infants <1 year of age, have a significantly increased mortality awaiting transplantation than older children. While overall mortality while awaiting heart transplantation in pediatric candidates has improved over time (Fig. 5.3c),[96] this era effect has not been observed in patients less than 1 year of age who continue to have a wait-list mortality of 19.9–27.7% over the past 10 years in the SRTR database. Over the same period of time, wait-list mortality in children 1–17 years of age decreased from 13.4% in 1997–1998 to 7.9% in 2005–2006, comparable to the decline in wait-list mortality in patients >18 years of age in the database. These findings suggest that in the face of a static rate of pediatric organ donation, improved medical management of pediatric heart transplant candidates over time has lowered wait-list mortality for older children, but not infants.

Patients with congenital heart disease may be listed for heart transplantation shortly after birth for several reasons: (1) they have a lesion felt not to be amenable to surgical repair or palliation; (2) they may have had an acutely unsuccessful surgical procedure and cannot be removed from intensive cardiac support; or (3) they have developed intractable cardiac symptomatology after what was an initially successful procedure(s). While some single-center experience has suggested pre-transplant mortality is comparable for congenital heart disease and cardiomyopathy patients,[101] both the PHTS (Fig. 5.3b) and SRTR[96] databases demonstrate that patients with congenital heart disease listed for heart transplantation have a significantly higher mortality while awaiting transplantation. The reasons for this increased mortality may in part be related to the larger proportion of infant heart transplant candidates who have congenital heart disease, in addition to the need for ventilatory or mechanical circulatory support in these patients who are listed for heart transplant after an acutely unsuccessful surgical procedure and who might also have substantial multi-organ dysfunction. While Mital et al.[102] did not find a relationship between pre-transplant mortality and duration from last cardiac surgery to listing for transplant, the PHTS experience with heart transplantation after the Fontan procedure[38] found a nearly 50% mortality in Fontan patients listed for transplantation less than 6 months after the procedure

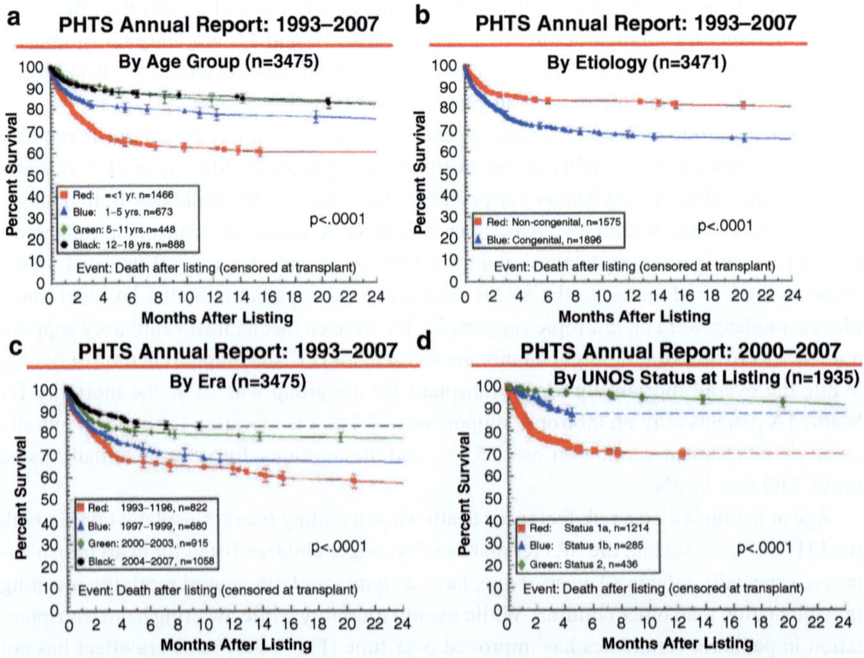

Fig. 5.3 Survival after listing for heart transplantation within the PHTS database from the 2008 annual report of the PHTS.[97] Patients are censored after transplantation. Panel A shows the significant differences in mortality while waiting among infant candidates compared to older children and adolescents. Panel B shows the significantly higher mortality prior to transplantation in patients with congenital heart disease compared to those with cardiomyopathy. Panel C shows the significant decrease in mortality prior to transplant in patients listed in the more recent eras. Panel D demonstrates the significantly increased mortality in pediatric patients listed as UNOS Status 1A urgency compared to Status 1B or 2

compared to over 90% survival in candidates whose Fontan was performed greater than 6 months before listing (Fig. 5.4). In addition, transplant candidates with congenital heart disease and with a past history of previous surgeries, blood transfusions, and utilization of human allograft material in their surgical repairs may develop antibodies to HLA antigens (presensitization).[103] These patients often will not be transplanted without a prospective compatible donor/recipient crossmatch which is associated with longer wait list times and higher pre-transplant mortality.[104]

A number of interventions have been proposed to reduce mortality in children awaiting heart transplantation. In infants these have included listing fetuses prior to birth,[105] the use of donors after declaration of cardio-circulatory death,[106] and ABO-incompatible transplantation.[107] ABO-incompatible transplantation is feasible in infants as they do not develop antibodies to ABO blood type for at least several months after birth. Increasing experience with ABO-incompatible infant heart transplantation[108,109] suggests no increased risk in mortality after transplantation in this group of patients, the development of “tolerance” to the mismatched blood group antigen in the recipient[110]

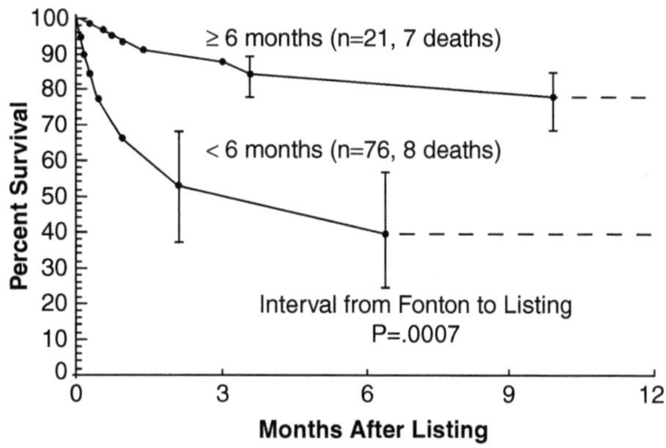

Fig. 5.4 Mortalitya mong patients with a previous Fontan procedure within the PHTSda tabase.[38]Pa tients listed less than 6 months after the Fontan procedure had a significantly higher mortality while awaiting transplantation

and perhaps an improvement in the likelihood of transplantation and reduction in wait-list mortality.[111] In older children, initial encouraging results have been achieved with immunosuppression protocols designed to permit transplantation of presensitized patients without a prospective compatible crossmatch.[112,113] Finally, the increasing use of VADs as a bridge to transplantation will likely provide more effective support and reduce mortality prior to transplantation. The recent availability of the Berlin Heart[88,114] in North America as well as Europe can offer VAD support to infants as small as 3.5 kg. Initial experience in the PHTS demonstrates substantial reductions in wait-list mortality in patients supported with VADs.[115] However, these results were not realized in patients listed for transplant with congenital heart disease, which was a risk factor for death after VAD insertion.

5.5 Outcomes of Heart Transplant Candidates with Congenital Heart Disease After Transplantation

Within the ISHLT database, the "half-life," or time after transplant at which 50% of heart transplant recipients die or require retransplantation is 15.7 years for infants less than 1 year of age; 15 years for children aged 1–10 years; 11.3 years for adolescents 11–17 years; and 10 years for patients greater than 18 years of age at time of transplantation.[4,5] Over the past 25 years, there has been a definite "era" effect in these databases as well; with improving short-term survival in the more recent eras. This same era effect has been noted in the PHTS, where significant improvement in survival has been observed both early and late after transplant (Fig. 5.5).[116]

A diagnosis of congenital heart disease is a risk factor for 1 year survival after heart transplantation in the pediatric and adult components of the ISHLT database.[4,5] Patients with congenital heart disease demonstrate a significantly poorer survival in both the PHTS

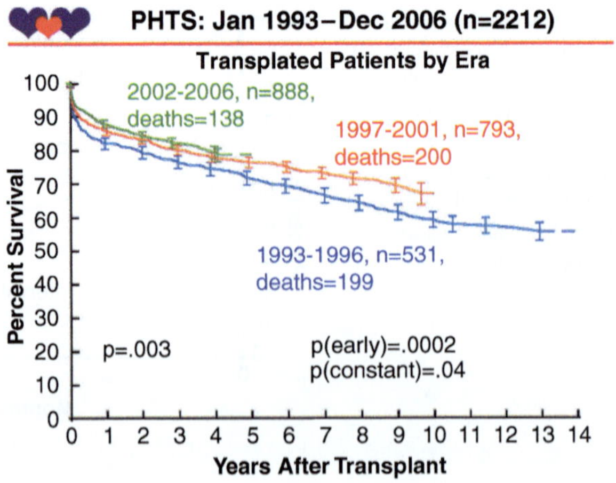

Fig. 5. 5 Theimprove menti n survival after transplantation in the recent era (2002–2006) compared to earlier eras in thePH TSda tabase.[116]A significant reduction in mortality has been observed not only in early survival, but in ongoing survival after transplantation

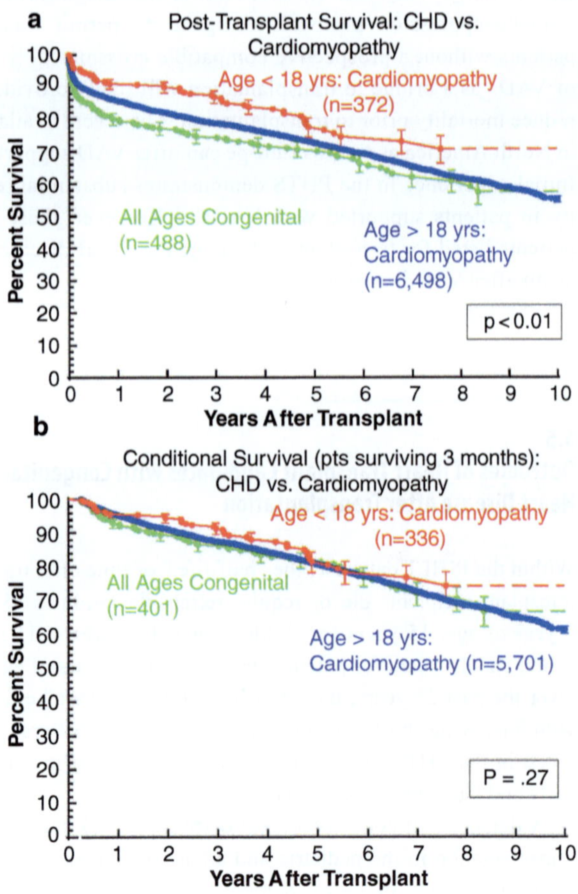

Fig. 5. 6 Ac omparisonof survival after transplantation for children and adults with congenital heart disease compared to children and adults transplanted for cardiomyopathy within the PHTS and CTRD databases.[6, 35]Pa nelA demonstrates that patients with congenital heart disease have significantly poorer survival after transplantation than do children transplanted for cardiomyopathy. Panel B demonstrates that survival is not significantly different between these groups among those patients who survive the first 3 months after transplantation

and CTRD databases (children and adults) after heart transplantation than patients transplanted for cardiomyopathy (Fig. 5.6a).[6] While large volume single centers have reported improvement in survival after heart transplantation for patients with congenital heart disease over time,[39,117] a similar era effect has not been observed within the PHTS database.[6] However, congenital heart disease only increases the risk of mortality immediately after transplant. As demonstrated in Fig. 5.6b from the PHTS/CTRD databases[6] and also observed in the ISHLT database,[5] both pediatric and adult patients transplanted for congenital heart disease who survive the first 3 months after transplant have outcomes no different than patients transplanted for cardiomyopathy.

The reasons that patients transplanted for congenital heart disease have higher early phase mortality are multifactorial. In Lamour's analysis of pediatric and adult congenital heart disease patients from the PHTS and CTRD databases[6] the significant risk factors for early phase mortality included older recipient age, increasing graft ischemic time, an interaction with donor age and ischemic time, and previous Fontan procedure. A poorer survival in patients with univentricular hearts transplanted after a Fontan procedure compared to those transplanted before a Fontan procedure has been observed in some single center studies[37,39] but not others.[36] A past history of a Fontan procedure was associated with an increased risk for death in the combined PHTS/CTRD analysis[6] of heart transplantation in *children and adults* with congenital heart disease. However, the survival after transplantation for a failed Fontan procedure in the PHTS database alone (patients transplanted at less than 18 years of age) was not significantly worse compared to patients transplanted for other congenital heart diseases.[38] Thus patients with a Fontan procedure who are transplanted as adults may represent an especially difficult subgroup.

Early reports from the heart transplant group at Columbia University in New York emphasized the surgical complexities of the heart transplant procedure in pediatric[118] and adult[119] patients with congenital heart disease, noting that the procedures were associated with longer ischemic times and increased perioperative bleeding. A need for pulmonary artery reconstruction has been specifically associated with an increased risk for mortality.[117] Challenging surgical reconstructions can be associated with prolongation of surgical implant times (warm ischemia) which may be more damaging to the allograft than the duration of transport time (cold ischemia).[120]

Two recent analyses by Davies[121,122] have explored the cumulative effect of risk factors on survival after pediatric heart transplantation. Davies' analysis of the UNOS database[121] noted that pretransplant renal failure (creatinine clearance less than 40 mL/min) was consistently predictive of poor outcome. In his analysis of the PHTS database[122] significant high risk criteria present at time of transplant for mortality after transplantation included: recipient age less than 1 month; need for ECMO or intra-aortic balloon pump; need for mechanical ventilation; previous sternotomy(ies); presensitization; and congenital heart disease. Pretransplant recipient characteristics *not predictive* of poor outcomes included recipient age 1 month to 1 year; location in an intensive care unit; need for inotropic support; UNOS status; history of renal insufficiency or pulmonary hypertension; or hypoalbuminemia. Interestingly, patients transplanted on an intra-aortic balloon pump or ECMO were at greater risk for death, but patients transplanted on a VAD were not, likely reflecting the superior support offered by VADs compared to other means of mechanical circulatory support.

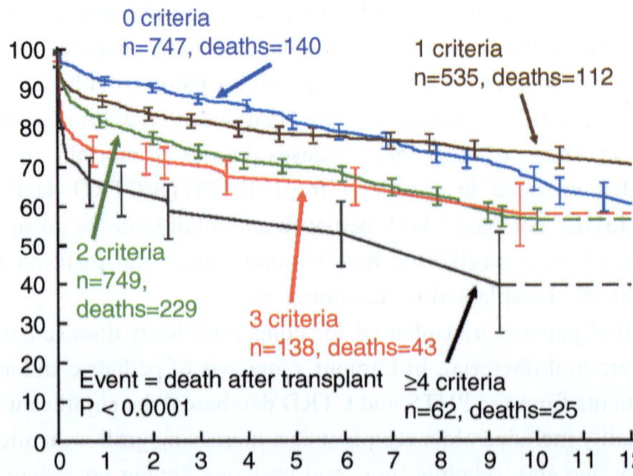

Fig. 5.7 The incremental impact of the presence of various high risk factors on survival after heart transplantation within the PHTS database.[122] Age less than 1 month, ECMO, mechanical ventilation, previous sternotomy(ies), presensitization, and diagnosis of congenital heart disease were identified as high risk factors for death after transplantation. One year survival exceeds 90% for patients with 0 risk factors and is less than 70% when 4 or more risk factors are present

Davies further noted additive detrimental effects on survival when patients had increasing numbers of these risk factors present at time of transplant. Figure 5.7[122] demonstrates that patients in the PHTS database with no high risk factors have a 1 year survival greater than 90% 1 year after transplant. The presence of one to 2 risk factors decreases one year survival to less than 90%; with 3 risk factors it drops to less than 80%; and with 4 or more risk factors it decrease to less than 70%. These findings underscore the effects of these comorbidities on outcomes in patients transplanted with congenital heart disease, especially neonatal candidates and/or patients transplanted after acutely unsuccessful surgical procedures. It is also notable that many of the risk factors associated with an increased risk of mortality after transplant are also associated with an increased risk for mortality in listed patients awaiting heart transplantation.

5.6 Concluding Remarks

Heart transplantation has evolved from a purely heroic therapy to, in some centers, the accepted final option for patients born with congenital heart disease. Overall outcomes for these patients appear in large multi-center registries to be poorer than those patients with cardiomyopathy and perhaps not improving over time. However, it should also be noted that the severity of illness prior to transplant in pediatric heart transplant recipients has also increased over time,[116] with an increasing proportion of pediatric heart transplants being performed on patients on ECMO, ventilators, inotropes, and/or with a history of renal insufficiency. The decision as to when patients with congenital heart should receive further conventional surgery versus heart transplantation is thus being continuously redefined. Heart transplantation as a therapy, like all other therapies, has its limitations. Viewing it as a therapy to be used in conjunction with other medical and surgical therapies, and not solely as a heroic therapy of last resort used only after all other options have failed, will likely maximize its effectiveness in patients with congenital heart disease.

References

1. Kantrowitz A, Haller JD, Joos H, Cerruti MM, Carstensen HE. Transplantation of the heart in an infant and an adult. *Am J Cardiol.*1968; 22:782–790.
2. Pennington DG, Sarafian J, Swartz M. Heart transplantation in children. *Heart Transplant.* 1985;4:441–445.
3. Starnes VA, Stinson EB, Oyer PE, Valantine H, Baldwin JC, Hunt SA, Shumway NE. Cardiac transplantation in children and adolescents. *Circulation.*1987; 76(supplV):V43–V47.
4. Kirk R, Edwards LB, Aurora P, Taylor DO, Christie J, Dobbels F, Kucheryavaya AY, Rahmel AO, Hertz MI. Registry of the International Society for Heart and Lung Transplantation: eleventh official pediatric heart transplantation report-2008. *J Heart Lung Transplant.* 2008;27:970–977.
5. Taylor DO, Edwards LB, Aurora P, Christie JD, Dobbels F, Kirk R, Rahmel AO, Kucheryavaya AY, Hertz MI. Registry of the International Society for Heart and Lung Transplantation: twenty-fifth official adult heart transplant report-2008. *J Heart Lung Transplant.*2008;2 7:943–956.
6. Lamour JM, Kanter KR, Naftel DC, Chrisant MR, Morrow WR, Clemson BS, Kirklin JK. The effect of age, diagnosis and previous surgery in 488 children and adults who undergo heart transplantation for congenital heart disease (abstract). *J Am Coll Cardiol.* 2005; 45:322A.
7. Chiavarelli M, Gundry SR, Razzouk AJ, Bailey LL. Cardiac transplantation for infants with hypoplastic left-heart syndrome. *JAMA.*1993; 270:2944–2947.
8. Backer CL, Zales VR, Harrison HL, Idriss FS, Benson DW, Mavroudis C. Intermediate term results of infant orthotopic cardiac transplantation from two centers. *J Thorac Cardiovasc Surg.*1991;101:826–832.
9. Canter CE, Spray TL, Huddleston CB, Moorhead S. Restrictive atrial communication as a determinant of outcome after cardiac transplantation for hypoplastic left heart syndrome. *Circulation.*1993;88(supplI I):II456–II460.
10. Canter CE, Naftel D, Caldwell R, Chinnock R, Pahl E, Frazier E, Kirklin J, Boucek M, Morrow WR. Survival and risk factors for death after cardiac transplantation in infants: a multi-institutional study. *Circulation.*1997; 96:227–231.
11. Ibrahim JE, Sweet SC, Flippin M, Dent C, Mendeloff E, Huddleston CB, Canter CE. Rejection is reduced in thoracic organ recipients when transplanted in the first year of life. *J Heart Lung Transplant.*2002;2 1:311–318.
12. Webber SA, Naftel DC, Parker J, Mulla N, Balfour I, Kirklin JK, Morrow WR. Late rejection episodes more than 1 year after pediatric heart transplantation: risk factors and outcomes. *J Heart Lung Transplant.*2003; 22:869–875.
13. Pahl E, Naftel DC, Kuhn MA, Shaddy RE, Morrow WR, Canter CE, Kirklin J. The impact and outcome of transplant coronary artery disease in a pediatric population: a 9 year multiinstitutional study. *J Heart Lung Transplant.*2005; 24:645–651.

14. Nicolas RT, Kort HW, Balzer DT, Trinkaus K, Dent CL, Hirsch R, Canter CE. Surveillance for transplant coronary artery disease in infant, child, and adolescent heart transplant recipients: an intravascular ultrasound study. *J Heart Lung Transplant.*2006; 25:921–927.
15. Mudge GH, Goldstein S, Addonizio LJ, Caplan A, Mancini D, Levine TB, Ritsch ME, Stevenson LW. Task Force 3: recipient guidelines/prioritization. 24th Bethesda conference: cardiac transplantation. *J Am Coll Cardiol.*1993; 22:21–31.
16. Costanzo MR, Augustine S, Bourge R, Bristow M, O'Connell JB, Driscoll D, Rose E. Selection and treatment of candidates for heart transplantation. *Circulation.* 1995;92: 3593–3612.
17. Jacobs ML, Blackstone EH, Bailey LL. Intermediate survival in neonates with aortic atresia: a multi-institutional study. *J Thorac Cardiovasc Surg.*1998; 116:417–431.
18. Jenkins PC, Flanagan MF, Jenkins KJ, Sargent JD, Canter CE, Chinnock RE, Vincent RN, Tosteson ANA, O'Connor GT. Survival analysis and risk factors for mortality in transplantation and staged surgery for hypoplastic left heart syndrome. *J Am Coll Cardiol.* 2000;36:1178–1185.
19. Jenkins PC, Flanagan MF, Sargent JD, Canter CE, Chinnock RE, Jenkins KJ, Vincent RN, O'Connor GT, Tosteson ANA. A comparison of treatment strategies for hypoplastic left heart syndrome using decision analysis. *J Am Coll Cardiol.* 2001;38:1181–1187.
20. Organ Procurement and Transplant Network (OPTN) website as of October 20, 2008. (http://www.OPTN.org).
21. Mahle WT, Spray TL, Wernovsky G, Gaynor JW, Clark BJ. Survival after reconstructive surgery for hypoplastic left heart syndrome. A 15-year experience from a single institution. *Circulation.*2000; 102(suppl II):III-146-41.
22. Azakie A, Merklinger SL, McCrindle BW, Van Arsdell GS, Lee K, Benson LN, Coles JG, Williams WG. Evolving strategies and improving outcomes of the modified Norwood procedure: a 10-year single-institution experience. *Ann Thorac Surg.*2001; 72:1349–1353.
23. Tweddell JS, Hoffman GM, Mussatto KA, Fedderly RT, Berger S, Jaquiss RD, Ghanayem NS, Frisbee SJ, Litwin SB. Improved survival of patients undergoing palliation of hypoplastic left heart syndrome: lessons learned from 115 consecutive patients. *Circulation.* 2002; 106(supplI):I82– I89.
24. Chrissant MRK, Naftel DC, Drummond-Webb J, Chinnock R, Canter CE, Boucek MM, Boucek RJ, Hallowell SC, Kirklin JK, Morrow WR. Fate of infants with hypoplastic left heart syndrome listed for cardiac transplantation: a multicenter study. *J Heart Lung Transplant.* 2005;24:576–582.
25. Canter CE, Shaddy RE, Bernstein D, Hsu DT, Chrisant MRK, Kirklin JK, Kanter KR, Higgins RSD, Blume ED, Rosenthal DN, Boucek MM, Uzark KC, Friedman AH, Young JK. Indications for heart transplantation in pediatric and congenital heart disease. An American Heart Association Scientific Statement. *Circulation.*2007; 115:658–676.
26. Linn JSL, McCrindle BW, Smallhorn JF, Golding F, Caldarone CA, Taketazu M, Jaeggi ET. Clinical features, management, and outcome of children with fetal and postnatal diagnoses of isomerism syndromes. *Circulation.*2005; 112:2454–2461.
27. Larsen RL, Eguchi JH, Mulla NF, Johnston JK, Fitts J, Kuhn MA, Razzouk AJ, Chinnock RE. Usefulness of cardiac transplantation in children with visceral heterotaxy (asplenic and polysplenic syndromes and single right-sided spleen with levocardia) and comparison of results with cardiac transplantation in children with dilated cardiomyopathy. *Am J Cardiol.* 2002;89:1275–1279.
28. Sarris GE, Giannopoulos NM, Tsoutsinos AJ et al. Results of surgery for Ebstein anomaly: a multicenter study from the European Congenital Heart Surgeons Association. *J Thorac Cardiovasc Surg.*2006; 132:50–57.
29. Shinebourne EA, Rigby ML, Carvalho JS. Pulmonary atresia with intact ventricular septum: from fetus to adult: congenital heart disease. *Heart.*2008; 94:1350–1357.

30. Guleserian KJ, Armsby LB, Thiagarajan RR, del Nido PJ, Mayer JE, Jr. Natural history of pulmonary atresia with intact ventricular septum and right-ventricle-dependent coronary circulation managed by the single-ventricle approach. *Ann Thorac Surg.* 2006;81: 2250–2257; discussion 2258.
31. Rychik J, Levy H, Gaynor JW, DeCampli WM, Spray TL. Outcome after operations for pulmonary atresia with intact ventricular septum. *J Thorac Cardiovasc Surg.* 1998;116: 924–931.
32. Ashburn DA, Blackstone EH, Wells WJ, Jonas RA, Pigula FA, Manning PB, Lofland GK, Williams WG, McCrindle BW. Determinants of mortality and type of repair in neonates with pulmonary atresia and intact ventricular septum. *J Thorac Cardiovasc Surg.* 2004;127: 1000–1008.
33. Glatz JA, Fedderly RT, Ghanayem NS, Twedell JS. Impact of mitral stenosis and aortic atresia on survival in hypoplastic left heart syndrome. *Ann Thorac Surg.*2008; 85:2057–2062.
34. Vida VL, Bacha EA, Larrazabal A, Gauvreau K, Dorfman AL, Marx G, Geva T, Marhsall AC, Pigula FA, Mayer JE, del Nido PJ, Fynn-Thompson F. Surgical outcome for patients with the mitral stenosis-aortic atresia variant of hypoplastic left heart syndrome. *J Thorac Cardiovasc Surg.*2008;135:339–346.
35. Hsu DT, Lamour JM, Canter CE. Heart diseases leading to pediatric heart transplantation: cardiomyopathies and congenital heart diseases. *Pediatric Heart Transplantation ISHLT Monograph.* Series 2, 2007, Elsevier, Philadelphia:1–17.
36. Jayakumar KA, Addonizio LJ, Kichuk-Chrisant MR et al. Cardiac transplantation after the Fontan or Glenn procedure. *J Am Coll Cardiol.*2004; 44:2065–2072.
37. Michielon G, Parisi F, Squitieri C, Carotti A, Gagliardi G, Pasquini L, Di Donato RM. Orthotopic heart transplantation for congenital heat disease: an alternative for high-risk Fontan candidates? *Circulation.*2003; 108(suppll I):II140–II149.
38. Bernstein D, Naftel D, Chin C et al. Outcome of listing for cardiac transplantation for failed Fontan: a multi-institutional study. *Circulation.*2006; 114:273–280.
39. Simmonds J, Burch M, Dawkins H, Tsang V. Heart transplantation after congenital heart surgery: improving results and future goals. *Eur J Cardiovasc Surg.*2008; 34:313–317.
40. Khairy P, Fernandes SM, Mayer JE, Triedman JK, Walsh EP, Lock JE, Landzberg MJ. Long-term survival, modes of death, and predictors of mortality in patients with Fontan surgery. *Circulation.*2008;1 17:85–92.
41. Fontan F, Kirklin JW, Fernandez G, Coast F, Naftel DC, Tritto F, Blackstone EH. Outcome after a "perfect" Fontan operation. *Circulation.*1990; 81:1520–1536.
42. Hraska V, Duncan BW, Mayer JE, Jr., Freed M, del Nido PJ, Jonas RA. Long-term outcome of surgically treated patients with corrected transposition of the great arteries. *J Thorac Cardiovasc Surg.*2005; 129:182–191.
43. Yoshimura N, Yamaguchi M, Oshima Y et al. Risk factors influencing early and late mortality after total cavopulmonary connection. *Eur J Cardiothorac Surg.*2001; 20:598–602.
44. Takeuchi K, McGowan FX, Jr., Bacha EA et al. Analysis of surgical outcome in complex double-outlet right ventricle with heterotaxy syndrome or complete atrioventricular canal defect. *Ann Thorac Surg.*2006; 82:146–152.
45. Dos L, Teruel L, Ferreira IJ et al. Late outcome of Senning and Mustard procedures for correction of transposition of the great arteries. *Heart.*2005 ;91:652–656.
46. Gatzoulis MA, Munk MD, Williams WG, Webb GD. Definitive palliation with cavopulmonary or aortopulmonary shunts for adults with single ventricle physiology. *Heart.* 2000; 83:51–57.
47. Hagler DJ. Palliated congenital heart disease. *Adolesc Med.*2001; 12:23–34.
48. Diller GP, Dimopoulos KD, Okonko D, Li W, Babu-Narayan SV, Broberg CS, Johansson B, Bouzas B, Mullen MJ, Poole-Wilson PA, Francis DP, Gatzoulis MA. Exercise intolerance in

adult congenital heart disease: comparative severity, correlates and prognostic implications. *Circulation*.2005; 112:828–835.
49. Gentles TL, Gauvreau K, Mayer JE, Fishberger SB, Burnett J, Colan SD, Newburger JW, Wernovsky G. Functional outcome after the Fontan operation: factors influencing late morbidity. *J Thorac Cardiovasc Surg*.1997; 114:392–403.
50. Driscoll DJ, Offord KP, Feldt RH, Schaff HV, Puga FJ, Danielson GK. Five-to fifteen-year follow-up after Fontan operation. *Circulation*.1992; 85:469–496.
51. Mancini DM, Eisen H, Kussmaul W, Mull R, Edmonds LH Jr, Wilson JR. Value of peak exercise oxygen consumption for optimal timing of cardiac transplantation in ambulatory patients with heart failure. *Circulation*.1991; 83:778–786.
52. Kao W, Jessup M. Exercise testing and exercise training in patients with congestive heart failure. *J Heart Lung Transplant*.1994; 13:S117–S121.
53. Aaronson KD, Mancini DM. Is percentage of predicted maximal exercise oxygen consumption a better predictor of survival than peak exercise oxygen consumption for patients with severe heart failure? *J Heart Lung Transplant*.1995: 14:81–89.
54. Stelken AM, Younis LT, Jennison SH, Miller DD, Miller LW, Shaw LJ, Kargl D, Chaitman BR. Prognostic value of cardiopulmonary exercise testing using percent achieved of predicted peak oxygen uptake for patients with ischemic and dilated cardiomyopathy. *J Am Coll Cardiol*. 1996;27:345–352.
55. O'Neill JO, Young JB, Pothier CE, Lauer MS. Peak oxygen consumption as a predictor of death in patients with heart failure receiving β-blockers. *Circulation*.2005; 111:2313–2318.
56. Miller LW. Listing criteria for cardiac transplantation: results of an American Society of Transplant Physicians-National Institutes of Health conference. *Transplantation*.1998; 66:947–951.
57. Ponikowski P, Francis DP, Piepoli MF, Davies LC, Chua TP, Davos CH, Florea V, Banasiak W, Poole-Wilson PA, Coats AJS, Anker SD. Enhanced ventilatory response to exercise in patients with chronic heart failure and preserved exercise tolerance. Marker of abnormal cardiorespiratory reflex control and predictor of poor prognosis. *Circulation*. 2001;103:967–972.
58. Wilson JR, Rayos G, Yeoh T et al. Dissociation between peak exercise oxygen consumption and hemodynamic dysfunction in potential heart transplant candidates. *J Am Coll Cardiol*. 1995;26:429–435.
59. Lund LH, Aaronson KD, Mancini DM. Validation of peak exercise oxygen consumption and the heart failure severity score for serial risk stratification in advanced heart failure. *Am J Cardiol*.2005;95 :734–741.
60. Aaronson KD, Schwartz JS, Chen T, Wong K, Goin JE, Mancini DM. Development and prospective validation of a clinical index to predict survival in ambulatory patients referred for cardiac transplant evaluation. *Circulation*.1997; 95:2660–2667.
61. Washington RL, van Gundy JC, Cohen C, Sondheimer HM, Wolfe RR. Normal aerobic and anaerobic exercise data in North American school-age children. *J Pediatr*. 1988;112:223–233.
62. Braden DS, Carroll JF. Normative cardiovascular responses to exercise in children. *Pediatr Cardiol*.1999;20 :4–10.
63. Fredriksen PM, Ingjer F, Nystad W, Thaulow E. A comparison of VO_{2peak} between patients with congenital heart disease and healthy subjects, all aged 8–17 years. *Eur J Appl Physiol*. 1999;80:409–416.
64. Giardini A, Hager A, Napoleone CP, Picchio FM. Natural history of exercise capacity after the Fontan operation: a longitudinal study. *Ann Thorac Surg*.2008; 85:818–822.
65. Paridon SM, Mitchell PD, Colan SD, Williams RV, Blafox A, Li JS, Margossian R, Mital S, Russell J, Rhodes J. A cross-sectional study of exercise performance during the first 2 decades of life after the Fontan operation. *J Am Coll Cardiol*.2 008;52:99–107.
66. Kamphuis M, Ottenkamp J, Vliegen HW, Vogels T, Zwinderman KH, Kamphuis RP, Verloove-Vanhorick SP. Health related quality of life and health status in adult survivors with previously operated complex congenital heart disease. *Heart*.200 2;87:356–362.

67. Hager A, Hess J. Comparison of health related quality of life with cardiopulmonary exercise testing in adolescents and adults with congenital heart disease. *Heart*.2005; 91:517–520.
68. McCrindle BW, Williams RV, Mitchell PD et al. Relationship of patient and medical characteristics to health status in children and adolescents after the Fontan procedure. *Circulation*. 2006;113:1123–1129.
69. Dimopoulos K, Okonko DO, Diller G-P, Broberg CS, Salukhe TV, Babu-Narayan SV, Li W, Uebing A, Bayne S, Wensel R, Piepoli MF, Poole-Wilson PA, Francis DP, Gatzoulis MA. Abnormal ventilatory response to exercise in adults with congenital heart disease relates to cyanosis and predicts survival. *Circulation*.2006; 113:2796–2802.
70. Diller G-P, Dimopoulos K, Okonko D, Uebing A, Broberg CS, Babu-Narayan S, Bayne S, Poole-Wilson PA, Sutton R, Francis DP, Gatzoulis MA. Heart rate response during exercise predicts survival in adults with congenital heart disease. *J Am Coll Cardiol*. 2006;48: 1250–1256.
71. del Nido PJ, Bailey LL, Kirklin JK. Surgical techniques in pediatric heart transplantation. *Pediatric Heart Transplantation ISHLT Monograph*. Series 2, 2007, Elsevier, Philadelphia: 83–102.
72. Cimato TR, Jessup M. Recipient selection in cardiac transplantation: contraindications and risk factors for mortality. *J Heart Lung Transplant*.2002 ;21:1 161–1173.
73. Gajarski RJ, Mosca RS, Ohye RG, Bove EL, Crowley DC, Custer JR, Moler FW, Valentini A, Kulik TJ. Use of extracorporeal life support as a bridge to pediatric cardiac transplantation. *J Heart Lung Transplant*.2003; 22(1):28–34.
74. Mehta U, Laks H, Sadeghi A, Marelli D, Odim J, Alejos J et al. Extracorporeal membrane oxygenation for cardiac support in pediatric patients. *Am Surg*.2000; 66(9):879–886.
75. Friedrich-Rust M, Koch C, Rentzsch A, Sarrazin C, Schwarz P, Herrmann E, Lindinger A, Sarrazin U, Poynard T, Schäfers, Zeuzem S, Abdul-Khaliq H. Noninvasive assessment of liver fibrosis in patients with Fontan circulation using transient elastography and biochemical fibrosis markers. *J Thorac Cardiovasc Surg*.2008; 135:560–567.
76. Lesser DB, Jeevanandam V, Furukawa S, Eisen H, Mather P, Silva P, Guy S, Foster CE. Simultaneous heart and kidney transplantation in patients with end-stage heart and renal failure. *Am J Transplant*.2001; 1:89–92.
77. Vremes E, Kirsch M, Houël, Legouvelo S, Benvenuti C, Aptecar E, Le Besnerais P, Lang P, Abbou C, Loisance D. Immunologic events and long-term survival after combined heart and kidney transplantation: 1 12-year single-center experience. *J Heart Lung Transplant*. 2001;20:1084–1091.
78. Porrett PM, Desai SS, Timmins KJ, Twomey CR, Sonnad SS, Olthoff KM. Combined orthotopic heart and liver transplantation: the need for exception status listing. *Liver Transplant*. 2004;10:1539–1544.
79. Huang J, Trinkaus K, Huddleston CB, Mendeloff EN, Spray TL, Canter CE. Recipient as well as donor characteristics are risk factors for primary graft failure after pediatric cardiac transplantation. *J Heart Lung Transplant*.2004; 23:716–722.
80. Kirklin JK, Naftel DC, Kirklin JW, Blackstone EH, White-Williams C, Bourge RC. Pulmonary vascular resistance and the risk of heart transplantation. *J Heart Lung Transplant*. 1988;7:331–336.
81. Bourge RC, Naftel DC, Costanzo-Nordin MR, Kirklin KD, Young JB, Kubo SH, Olivari MT, Kasper EK. Pretransplantation risk factors for death after heart transplantation: a multiinstitutional study. *J Heart Lung Transplant*.1993; 12:549–562.
82. Bando K, Konishi H, Komatsu K, del Nido PJ, Francalancia NA, Hardesty RL, Griffith BP, Armitage JM. Improved survival following pediatric heart transplantation in high-risk patients. *Circulation*.1993;88: II218–II223.
83. Murali S, Kormos RL, Uretsky BF, Schechte D, Reddy PS, Denys BG, Armitage JM, Hardesty RL, Griffith BP. Preoperative pulmonary hemodynamics and early mortality after

orthotopic cardiac transplantation: the Pittsburgh experience. *Am Heart J.* 1993; 126:896–904.
84. Zales VR, Pahl E, Backer CL, Crawford S, Mavroudis C, Benson DW. Pharmacologic reduction of pretransplantation pulmonary vascular resistance predicts outcome after pediatric heart transplantation. *J Heart Lung Transplant.* 1993;12:965–973.
85. Gajarski RJ, Towbin JA, Bricker JT, Radovancevic B, Frazier OH, Price JK, Schowengerdt KO, Denfield SW. Intermediate follow-up of pediatric heart transplant recipients with elevated pulmonary vascular resistance index. *J Am Coll Cardiol.* 1994;23:1682–1687.
86. Adatia I, Perry S, Landzberg M, Moore P, Thompson JE, Wessel DL. Inhaled nitric oxide and hemodynamic evaluation of patients with pulmonary hypertension before transplantation. *J Am Coll Cardiol.* 1995;25:1656–1664.
87. Hughes Ml, Kleinert S, Keogh A, Macdonald P, Wilkinson JL, Weintraub RG. Pulmonary vascular resistance and reactivity in children with end-stage cardiomyopathy. *J Heart Lung Transplant.* 2000;19:701–704.
88. Gandhi SK, Huddleston CB, Balzer DT, Epstein DJ, Boschert TA, Canter CE. Biventricular assist devices as a bridge to heart transplantation in small children. *Circulation.* 2008;118(suppl1):S89–S93.
89. Chen JM, Davies RR, Mital SR, Mercando ML, Addonizio LJ, Pinney SP, Hsu DT, Lamour JM, Quaegebeur JM, Mosca RS. Trends and outcomes in transplantation for complex congenital heart disease: 1984 to 2004. *Ann Thorac Surg.* 2004;78:1352–1361.
90. Lamour JM, Hsu DT, Kichuk MR, Galantowicz ME, Quaegebeur JM, Addonizio LJ. Regression of pulmonary arteriovenous malformations following heart transplantation. *Pediatr Transplant.* 2000;4:280–284.
91. Kanter KR, Vincent RN, Raviele AA. Importance of acquired systemic-to-pulmonary collaterals in the Fontan operation. *Ann Thorac Surg.* 1999;68:969–975.
92. Krishnan US, Lamour DT, Hsu DT et al. Management of aortopulmonary collaterals in children following cardiac transplantation for complex congenital heart disease. *J Heart Lung Transplant.* 2004;23:948–953.
93. Cochrane AD, Adams DH, Radley-Smith R, Khaghni A, Yacoub MH. Heterotopic heart transplantation for elevated pulmonary vascular resistance in pediatric patients. *J Heart Lung Transplant.* 1995;14:296–301.
94. Foerster SR, Gauvreau K, McElhinney DB, Geva T. Importance of totally anomalous pulmonary venous connection and postoperative pulmonary vein stenosis in outcomes of heterotaxy syndrome. *Pediatr Cardiol.* 2008;29:536–544.
95. Graziano JN, Heidelberger KP, Ensing GJ, Gomez CA, Ludomirsky A. The influence of a restrictive atrial septal defect on pulmonary vascular morphology in patients with hypoplastic left heart syndrome. *Pediatr Cardiol.* 2002;23:146–151.
96. Mahle WT, Vincent RN. Analysis of heart transplant waitlist mortality for children (abstract). *Circulation.* 2008;118(suppl 2):S964.
97. Pediatric Heart Transplant Study Annual Report. November 1, 2008.
98. Renlund DG, Taylor DO, Kfoury AG, Shaddy RS. New UNOS rules: historical background and implications for transplantation management. *J Heart Lung Transplant.* 1999; 18:1065–1070.
99. Kirklin JK, Naftel DC, Caldwell RL, Pearce FB, Bartlett H, Rusconi P, White-Williams C, Robinson BV. Should status II patients be removed from the pediatric heart transplant waiting list? A multi-institutional study. *J Heart Lung Transplant.* 2006;25:271–275.
100. Almond C, Thiagarajan R, Piercey G, Gauvreau K, Bastardi H, Singh TP. Waitlist mortality among children listed for heart transplantation in the United States. (abstract). Pediatric Academic Societies. *Pediatric Research.* 2008.
101. Rosenthal DN, Dubin AM, Chin C, Falco D, Gamberg P, Bernstein D. Outcome while awaiting heart transplantation in children: a comparison of congenital heart disease and cardiomyopathy. *J Heart Lung Transplant.* 2000;19:751–755.
102. Mital S, Addonizio LJ, Lamour JM, Hsu DT. Outcome of children with end-stage congenital heart disease waiting for cardiac transplantation. *J Heart Lung Transplant.* 2003;22:147–153.

103. Shaddy RE, Fuller TC. The sensitized pediatric heart transplant candidate: causes, consequences, and treatment options. *Pediatr Transplant.* 2005;9:208–214.
104. Feingold B, Bowman P, Zeevi A, Girnita AL, Quivers ES, Miller SA, Webber SA. Survival in allosensitized children after listing for cardiac transplantation. *J Heart Lung Transplant.* 2007;26:565–571.
105. Pollock-BarZiv SM, McCrindle BW, West LJ, Dipchand AI. Waiting before birth: outcomes after fetal listing for heart transplantation. *Am J Transplant.* 2008;8:412–18.
106. Boucek MM, Mashburn C, Dunn SM, Frizell R, Edwards L, Pietra B, Campbell D. Pediatric heart transplantation after declaration of cardiocirculatroy death. *N Eng J Med.* 2008;359:709–714.
107. West LJ, Pollock-BarZiv, Dipchand AI et al. ABO-incompatible heart transplantation in infants. *N Engl J Med.* 2001;344:793–800.
108. Roche SL, Burch M, O'Sullivan J, Wallis J, Parry G, Kirk R, Elliot M, Shaw N, Flett J, Hamilton JRL, Hasan A. Multicenter experience of ABO-incompatible pediatric cardiac transplantation. *Am J Transplant.* 2008;8:208–215.
109. Patel ND, Weiss ES, Scheel J, Cameron DE, Vricella LA. ABO-incompatible heart transplantation in infants: analysis of the United Network for Organ Sharing database. *J Heart Lung Transplant.* 2008;27:1085–1089.
110. Fan X, Ang A, Pollock-BarZiv SM, Dipchand AI, Ruiz P, Wilson G et al. Donor-specific B-cell tolerance after ABO-incompatible infant heart transplant. *Nat Med.* 2004; 10:1227–1233.
111. West LJ, Karamlow T, Dipchand AI, Pollock BarZiv SM, Coles JG, McCrindle BW. Impact on outcomes after listing and transplantation, of a strategy to accept ABO blood group-incompatible donor hearts for neonates and infants. *J Thorac Cardiovasc Surg.* 2006; 131:455–461.
112. Holt DB, Lublin DM, Phelan DR, Boslaugh SE, Gandhi SK, Huddleston CB, Saffitz JE, Canter CE. Mortality and morbidity in presensitized pediatric heart transplant recipients with a positive donor crossmatch utilizing perioperative plasmapheresis and cytolytic therapy. *J Heart Lung Transplant.* 2007;26:876–882.
113. Pollock-BarZiv SM, den Hollander N, Ngan BY, Kantor P, McCrindle B, Dipchand AI. Pediatric heart transplantation in human leukocyte antigen sensitized patients: evolving management and assessment of intermediate-term outcomes in a high-risk population. *Circulation.* 2007;116(suppl I):I172–I178.
114. Malaisrie SC, Pelletier MP, Yun JJ, Sharma K, Timek TA, Rosenthal DN, Wright GE, Robbins RC, Reitz BA. Pneumatic paracorporeal ventricular assist device in infants and children: initial Stanford experience. *J Heart Lung Transplant.* 2008;27:173–177.
115. Blume ED, Naftel DC, Bastardi HJ, Duncan BW, Kirklin JK, Webber SA. Pediatric Heart Transplant Study Investigators. Outcomes of children bridged to heart transplantation with ventricular assist devices: a multi-institutional study. *Circulation.* 2006;113:2313–2319.
116. Naftel DC, Kirklin JK, Hsu DT, Blume ED, Webber SA, Morrow WR, Canter CE. Pediatric heart transplantation: 14 years of improving results illustrated by patient specific predictions (abstract). *J Heart Lung Transplant.* 2008;27:S253.
117. Chen JM, Davies RR, Mital SA, Mercando ML, Addonizio LJ, Pinney SP, Hsu DT, Lamour JM, Quaegebeur JM, Mosca RS. Trends and outcomes in transplantation for complex congenital heart disease: 1984–2004. *Ann Thorac Surg.* 2004;78:1352–1361.
118. Hsu DT, Quaegebeur JM, Michler RE, Smith CR, Rose EA, Kichuk MR, Gersony WM, Douglas JF, Addonizio LJ. Heart transplantation in children with congenital heart disease. *J Am Coll Cardiol.* 1995;26:743–749.
119. Lamour JL, Addonizio LJ, Galantowicz ME, Quaegebeur JM, Mancini DM, Kichuk MR, Benizminovitz A, Michler RE, Weinberg A, Hsu DT. Outcomes after orthotopic cardiac transplantation in adults with congenital heart disease. *Circulation.* 1999;100(suppl II):II200–II205.
120. Banner NR, Thomas HL, Curnow E, Hussey JC, Rogers CA, Bonser RS. The importance of cold and warm ischemia for survival after heart transplantation. *Transplantation.* 2008;86:542–547.

121. Davies RR, Russo MJ, Mital S, Martens TM, Sorabella RS, Hong KN, Gelijns AC, Moskowitz AJ, Quaegebeur JM, Mosca RS, Chen JM. Predicting survival among high-risk pediatric cardiac transplant recipients: an analysis of the United Network for Organ Sharing database. *J Thorac Cardiovasc Surg*. 2008;135:147–155.
122. Davies RR, Chen JM, Naftel DC, Boyle G, Zangwill S, Gararski R, Robinson B, Kirk R, Hsu D, Blume E. The impact of high-risk criteria on mortality following heart transplantation in children: a multi-institutional study (abstract). *J Heart Lung Transplant*. 2008;27: S255–S256.

Right Ventricular Failure in Congenital HeartD isease

6

Luis Antonio Altamiraa nd Andrew N. Redington

6.1 Introduction

It is not so long ago that the right ventricle was considered very much secondary to the left ventricle, in terms of both its influence on the normal circulation, and its impact on outcomes in acquired heart disease. The past two decades however, have seen a remarkable change in our understanding of its role. Fundamental to the normal circulation, the influence of heart–lung interactions, electro–mechanical interactions, and right–left heart interactions, have all been implicated as therapeutic targets in different forms of heart disease. Consequently, the important role of right ventricular dysfunction in determining the outcome of a variety of "left heart" diseases is now established. For example, it is now known that survival in dilated left ventricular cardiomyopathy is markedly influence by the co-existence of right ventricular dysfunction.[1]

In congenital heart disease, we have been much more aware of the importance of right ventricular dysfunction, particularly within the spectrum of heart failure syndromes associated with structural anomalies of the heart and their surgical treatment. Nonetheless, our understanding of the role of right ventricular dysfunction, the mechanisms of its pathophysiology, and ways in which it may be treated, are all continuing to evolve.

In this chapter we will review the current state of knowledge of the role of right ventricular dysfunction in the outcomes of congenital heart disease, using specific examples asill ustrations.

6.2 Formation and Origins of the Right Ventricle

It is beyond the scope of this chapter to discuss the development of the heart in any great detail, but we now know that the left and right ventricles are formed from cells within the

L.A.A ltamira(✉)
Pediatric Cardiology, The Hospital for Sick Children,
UniversityofT orontoSc hoolof M edicine, Toronto, Ontario, Canada

R.E. Shaddy (ed.), *Heart Failure in Congenital Heart Disease*,
DOI: 10.1007/978-1-84996-480-7_6, © Springer-Verlag London Limited 2011

developing embryo forming the first and second heart field respectively.[2] The migration, proliferation, and differentiation of these cells is closely regulated by specific transcription factors within the developing ventricular mass and are quite specific to each ventricle and its progenitors.[3] It would be surprising therefore, particularly given their markedly different roles, if the function of the right and left ventricular myocardium was not discernibly different at a structural, biochemical and physiologic level. Interestingly, such differences have been difficult to discern, even in experimental preparations. A faster twitch speed, and velocity of shortening, has been shown in myofibers from the normal right ventricle compared with the normal left ventricle,[4] but evidence for the right ventricle being the "weaker" ventricle is lacking. Indeed, as we will discuss below, despite the dogma, it appears that changing geometry and other epiphenomena (e.g. tricuspid valve function) are far greater predictors of right ventricular decline, than intrinsic myocyte contractile dysfunction, at least in the early to mid-term follow up of many congenital anomalies.

6.3 Anatomy and Geometry of the Right Ventricle

The right ventricle is a tripartite structure[5] formed by an inlet, an apical trabecular component, and an outlet portion. The inlet extends from the atrioventricular junction to the distal attachments of the tricuspid valve, with its chordae tendinae and papillary muscles characteristically inserting into the apex and septal surface of the right ventricle. The apical component is coarsely trabeculated, with its most obvious muscle bar being the moderator band, an extension of the septomarginal trabeculation that forms a strap like structure along the septal surface. The septomarginal trabeculation itself divides into anterior and posterior limbs beyond which forms the subpulmonary infundibulum. Unlike its left ventricular counterpart, there is no fibrous continuity between the inlet and outlet valve, the tricuspid and pulmonary valves being separated by a ventriculo-infundibular fold formed from the inner curvature of the heart. Consequently, the pulmonary valve sits on a complete muscular sleeve, the subpulmonary infundibulum.[6]

The histological arrangement of the ventricular mass remains a source of some debate with different theories regarding the continuity of muscle fibers and bands.[7–8] The detailed dissections of Sanchez-Quintana, and Anderson,[9] (Fig. 6.1) are the most compelling however. The normal right ventricle has two layers of myofibers, a subepicardial oblique and a subendocardial longitudinal layer. This is somewhat different from the left ventricle, which has an interposing circumferential middle layer, and perhaps forms the basis for the very different patterns of contraction (the right ventricle shortens largely in its long axis, the left ventricle shortens largely in its short axis). It is important to note however, that the subepicardial oblique myofibers are shared by the two ventricles. Indeed, it is possible to trace fibers extending from the right ventricular outflow tract, continuously to the left ventricular apex. This clearly sets the scene for myocardial cross talk, as one of the ways in which the right and left heart structures interact physiologically, and in disease (see below).

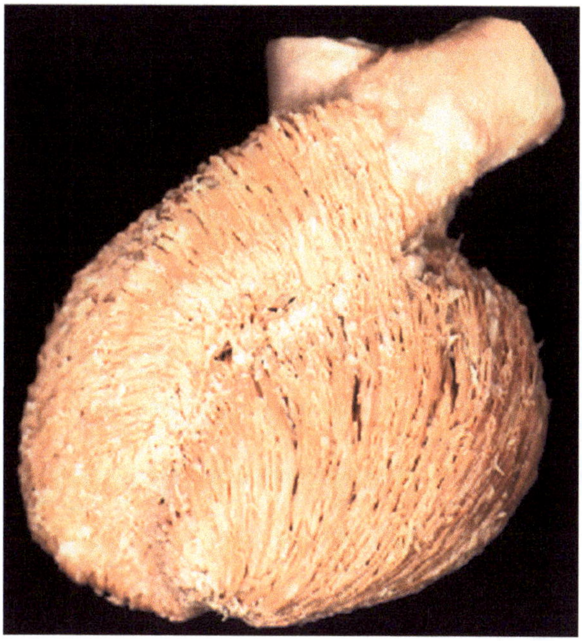

Fig.6. 1 Dissections howing the superficial myofibers from a normal heart. Note how individual bundles are continuous from the right ventricular outflow tract to the left ventricular apex, setting the scene for myocardial cross-talk as a mode of ventricular–ventricular interaction (See text for details. Image reproduced with permission ofProf.R HA nderson)

6.4 Normal Right Ventricular Physiology

The right ventricular output must be the same as the left ventricular output, give or take some allowance for small collateral circulations. However, because of the unique characteristics of the pulmonary vascular bed, the right ventricle is able to generate the same cardiac output at approximately one fifth of the energy cost of the left ventricle. Consequently the two ventricles have markedly different pressure volume relationships.[10]

6.4.1 Normal Right Ventricular Pressure Volume Relations

An understanding of the fundamental characteristics of right ventricle contractile physiology is important when assessing the impact of disease. Unlike the square wave pumping action of the left ventricle, whereby its pressure volume relationship is square or rectangular with clearly defined periods of isovolumic contraction and relaxation, the right ventricle has a quite different characteristic. Because of the low hydrolic impedance within the pulmonary vascular bed, the period of isovolumic contraction is brief and ejection from the ventricle, into the pulmonary artery, occurs early during pressure rise. Most importantly, much of right ventricular ejection, in health, occurs during pressure decline. After peak right ventricular pressure is reached, right ventricular volume continues to fall (ejection into the pulmonary artery continues to occur) as right ventricular pressure is falling. This phenomenon was originally suggested by the discovery of the hangout period, described by Shaver et al.[11] This is defined as a time delay between the onset of pressure decline in the right ventricle, and the timing of pulmonary valve closure. The correlate of this, in terms of its pressure volume curve, is that of an overall triangular or trapezoidal appearance with ejection from the right ventricle occurring during pressure rise and pressure fall.

While this is energetically efficient in the normal circulation, it is not a particularly robust system. Compared with the left ventricle, the right ventricle is several-fold more sensitive to changes in its afterload.[12] Indeed, a small rise in right ventricular afterload can lead to a rapid and linear decline in stroke volume and therefore cardiac output. While adaptation can occur with time, acute pulmonary hypertension is particularly poorly tolerated by the normal right ventricle, which explains the high mortality of conditions such as acute massive pulmonary embolism, for example.[13] Rapid right ventricular dilatation and reduced cardiac output leads to a reciprocal change in left ventricular filling and a vicious spiral of decline. This biventricular interaction is clearly adverse, but there are many beneficial left–right heart interactions that need to be understood before adverse situations can bedi scussed.

6.4.2 Right–Left Heart Interactions

As discussed above, the anatomy, geometry, and shared myocardium and pericardium, would all make the lack of right–left heart interactions more surprising than their existence. Indeed, there is substantial evidence to suggest that such interactions are fundamental to normal biventricular physiology. For example, it has been estimated that 30–40% of the mechanical work formed on the right side of the circulation, is a direct consequence of left ventricular contraction. This was confirmed in elegant studies of electrically isolated but mechanically contiguous hearts, reported by Damiano et al.[14] In their experiments, they showed that the very action of left ventricular contraction (in the absence of any electrical or direct mechanical stimulation of the right ventricle) lead to right ventricular shortening, and ejection from the right ventricle into the pulmonary artery. This phenomenon has been confirmed in a more direct way by Hoffman et al.[15] In their experiments, they removed the entire right ventricular free wall myocardium and replaced it with an artificial patch. They showed that left ventricular contraction led to generation of a substantial right ventricular stroke volume, even in the absence of right ventricular myocardium. Interestingly in this latter experiment, as the artificial right ventricle was enlarged, not only did right ventricular output fall, but there was also a fall in left ventricular output. These studies could not answer the question as to whether this was a series effect (low output from the right ventricle leading to low output of the left ventricle) or whether this was a parallel affect, whereby there was a direct and adverse influence of right heart dilatation on intrinsic left ventricular mechanics. To answer this, we studied this in a series of experiments in pigs.[16] Using biventricular conductance catheters, we were able to show that acute right heart dilatation immediately modified left ventricular intrinsic contractility as measured by preload recruitable stroke work and end systolic elastance. These affects were abrogated, but not abolished, by release of the pericardium, suggesting that this effect was largely a geometric interaction when the pericardium was closed, but almost certainly a cross talk phenomenon (because of shared myofibers), when the pericardium is open.

It has therefore become increasingly apparent, that it is spurious to examine the pathophysiology of isolated left ventricular or right ventricular disease, as disease in one ventricle one clearly modifies the function of the other. This also has important implications for potential therapies. Techniques directed toward improving performance of one side of the heart are likely to have beneficial effects on the contralateral side, and vice versa. Some of these concepts will be expanded upon in the subsequent sections.

6.5 Biventricular Interactions in "Right Heart Diseases"

6.5.1 The Pressure Loaded Right Ventricle

Primary pulmonary hypertension has traditionally been considered to be a uniquely right heart disease. While this is certainly the case in the earlier evolution of its pathophysiology, there are important biventricular consequences as the condition progresses. As discussed above, the right ventricle is particularly afterload sensitive, but when slowly increased, afterload increase in the form of progressive pulmonary hypertension may be tolerated remarkably well for many years. There is therefore a preclinical stage of pulmonary hypertension that is associated with modified pressure volume relationships, increasing right ventricular power, and normal cardiac output, despite substantial increases in pulmonary vascular resistance. This adaptive phase has been described both in animal models and in humans.[17–18]

As the pulmonary vascular resistance continues to rise, then right ventricular failure ensues. In primary pulmonary hypertension, this is usually at a point where the pulmonary vascular resistance substantially exceeds that of the systemic vascular resistance. In congenital heart diseases, the situation is more complex. In the Eisenmenger atrial septal defect, failure is somewhat earlier than with the Eisenmenger ventricular septal defect or arterial duct. This is not soley related to the additional, long-standing, right ventricular volume load associated with an atrial septal defect. As with primary pulmonary hypertension, the ventriculopulmonary circuit is "closed." Thus, the right ventricle in Eisenmenger ASD and primary pulmonary hypertension, is solely exposed to the pulmonary vascular resistance, which is often greater than the systemic vascular resistance. In the Eisenmenger VSD and ductus arteriosus, the right ventricle is exposed not only to the pulmonary vascular resistance, but also to the lower systemic vascular resistance. The ability therefore to shunt right to left across these lesions substantially reduces the hemodynamic burden on the right ventricle and improves survival,[19] albeit at the cost of earlier cyanosis in these patients.

Returning however, to the situation in primary pulmonary hypertension or the Eisenmenger ASD, ultimately the right ventricular myocardium will fail in the face of an inexorable rise in pulmonary vascular impedance. Failure is characterized by right ventricular dilatation, with an increasing end diastolic volume and end systolic volume. This sets the scene for the geometric biventricular interaction discussed above. As the right ventricle dilates, the left ventricle will be impaired, both in terms of its systolic shortening, and its diastolic filling.[20] This phenomenon of reduced early diastolic filling is well recognized in primary pulmonary hypertension, associated with right ventricular failure. This is not simply a geometric interaction however. Fundamental to this pathophysiology, is increased duration of right ventricular contraction.[20] A prolongation of right ventricular systole leads to persistent tension within the septum, interfering with early rapid filling of the left ventricle (Fig. 6.2). It is important to differentiate this from the characteristically decreased ejection time[21] into the pulmonary artery however. Increased right ventricular contraction time is evidenced by the prolongation of the duration of tricuspid incompetence, with its resultant shortening of diastolic filling time. Consequently, the right, and left, diastolic filling time (and therefore filling volume and stroke volume) is remarkably heart rate dependent. As the heart rate increases, there is a reduction in diastolic filling time, further reducing the ability of the left ventricle to fill. This pathophysiology has been beautifully demonstrated in cardiac magnetic resonance studies of patients with primary pulmonary hypertension.[22] Interestingly, the total stroke volume in the study patients was less dependent on right ventricular dilatation, and more associated with decrease left ventricular end diastolic volume, albeit as a secondary consequence of right ventricular dysfunction. Furthermore the stroke volume was also highly dependent on heart rate. The systolic: diastolic ratio (the S:D ratio) has recently been proposed as a simply measured

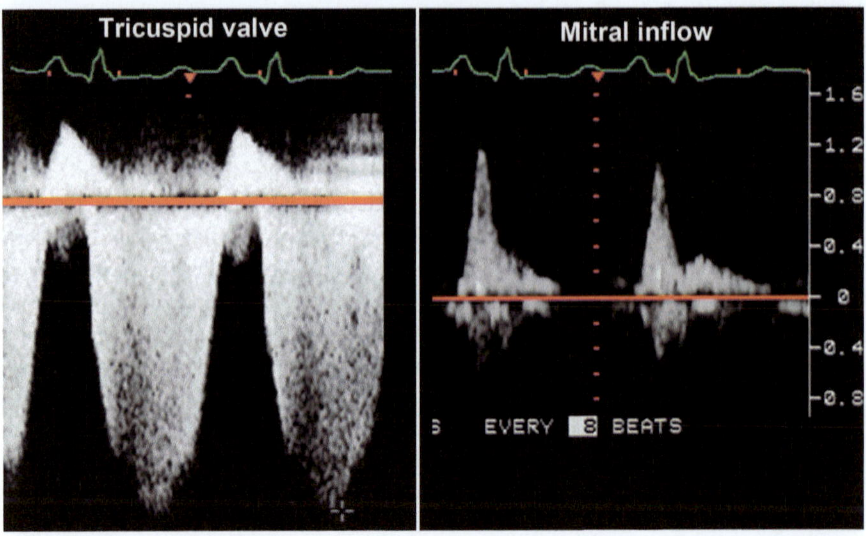

Fig. 6.2 Doppler recordings from a patient with severe pulmonary hypertension. Despite shortened ejection time into the pulmonary artery, the tricuspid valve regurgitation trace (*left panel*) shows that right ventricular contraction is markedly prolonged. While this clearly limits the time available for right ventricular filling, it also interferes with left ventricular filling. Persistent tension in the septum effectively abolishes early rapid filling through the mitral valve (*right panel*) there being exclusively atrial systolic flow

non invasive correlate of this physiology. In children with pulmonary hypertension, a higher S:D ratio is associated with worse survival.[23]

Consequently, avoidance of tachycardia, and relief of right ventricular afterload (pulmonary vasodilation) should be the aims of treatments in patients with primary pulmonary hypertension or Eisenmenger atrial septal defect.[24,25] While, paradoxically, creation of an atrial septal defect or PFO can modify the course of disease for patients with primary pulmonary hypertension, it is flawed as a treatment in terms of fundamental pathophysiology. Clearly an atrial septal defect may allow right-to-left shunting under these circumstances, increasing left ventricular preload at the expense of cyanosis but does little to affect the intrinsic drivers of right ventricular dysfunction and ultimate failure. Consequently, the outcome for patients with primary pulmonary hypertension, even in the presence of a naturally occurring, or artificially created atrial communication, is much worse than the Kaplan–Meier curve for Eisenmenger ductus arteriosus or VSD.[19] This begs the question as to whether improved survival might be associated with conversion of the physiology of primary pulmonary hypertension, to that of an Eisenmenger duct. In a small proof of principle study in children with primary pulmonary hypertension, this concept was explored surgically by creating an aortopulmonary window (Potts shunt) in children with right heart failure secondary to primary pulmonary hypertension. While not without risk, and clearly requiring wider experience before being offered as an established therapy, children undergoing this procedure had an improved quality of life and exercise performance.[25]

6.5.2 Right Ventricular Volume Overload

In congenital heart disease, the commonest form of persistent right ventricular volume overload is seen in patients after repair of tetralogy of Fallot. While previously considered to be a benign residua of successful surgery, it is now recognized that chronic pulmonary regurgitation with its secondary effects on right ventricular size, contractile performance, and mechanoelectric interactions, represent the largest burden, and commonest cause of symptoms in these patients.[26] We cannot discuss the determinants of pulmonary incompetence, and its treatment in detail, but we will discuss the biventricular implications of right heart dilatation under the circumstances.

The last decade or so has seen a gradual emergence of our understanding of biventricular disease in tetralogy of Fallot. Although most likely driven primarily by the effects of pulmonary regurgitation on the right ventricle, it has become clear that there is a loose, but linear, relationship between right ventricular dysfunction and left ventricular ejection fraction under these circumstances.[27] Furthermore, right ventricular dilation associated with overt left ventricular dysfunction is associated with poorer survival in the long-term follow up of adult patients.[28]

The exact mechanisms of this biventricular interaction are yet to be fully described, but include geometric, electrophysiologic, and mechanoelectric interactions. For example, we have recently confirmed that a significant geometric interaction occurs. In patients undergoing pulmonary valve replacement, not only was there an improvement in right ventricular ejection fraction, associated with reverse remodeling of the right ventricle, but there was a concomitant improvement in left ventricular ejection fraction.[29] This appeared to be relatively independent of other changes, such as QRS duration change, etc. Nonetheless there is also evidence that electrical incoordination may be a driver of this biventricular interaction. In an excellent study from the Calabro laboratory,[30] it was shown using tissue Doppler analysis that a marked incoordination between the onset of contraction of the two ventricles was associated with worse exercise performance and a greater propensity to ventricular arrhythmia. This interventricular dyssynchrony is a somewhat different concept to the more usual intraventricular dyssynchrony treated by biventricular pacing in adults with acquired heart disease. Nonetheless, it may be equally amenable to mechanoelectric interventions. Biventricular pacing has an evolving role in the treatment of many congenital heart diseases, but may be particularly useful under the circumstances of interventricular dyssynchrony. As an example of this, we recently reported remarkable functional improvement following biventricular pacing for interventricular, and septal, dyssynchrony after tetralogy of Fallot repair.[31] Clearly more work is required before guidelines and expectations for this therapy can be defined, but this is an exciting area of future research.

6.5.3 The Systemic Right Ventricle in a Biventricular Circulation

It is perhaps this area where there has been most confusion regarding the intrinsic nature of the right ventricular myocardium, and its ability to maintain a systemic cardiac output in the long-term. While it is true that almost every study of exercise performance, or myocardial functional performance, is able to demonstrate marked abnormalities compared with normal, it may well be that pure myocardial failure is relatively unusual as a cause of symptoms in this group of patients.

Taking the Mustard and Senning population as an example, the reduced right ventricular stroke volume characteristically seen with provocative testing (dobutamine stress, exercise) has often been ascribed to right ventricular dysfunction. While it would be difficult to deny the presence of abnormal right ventricular shortening in the majority of these patients, there is evidence that the mechanism for reduced stroke volume in these patients may lay elsewhere. Indeed, using a conductance catheter analysis to separate out the load dependent and load independent functional characteristics of the circulation, we have shown that the reduced stroke volume in these patients appears unrelated to intrinsic myocardial responses, under the circumstances of dobutamine stress.[32] Right ventricular contractility, relaxation characteristics, ventriculo-vascular coupling, and diastolic stiffness all responded appropriately to dobutamine stress. What was abnormal however was the unchanged rate of ventricular filling, despite a rapid and marked increase in heart rate. Under normal circumstances, the chronotropic effects of dobutamine are mirrored by a concomitant rise in ventricular filling rate. The consequence of an unchanged filling rate under these circumstances is clear. As the diastolic filling time reduces, a fixed rate of ventricular filling will lead to a fall in the absolute volume of ventricular filling, and therefore stroke volume (Fig. 6.3). The pathophysiology of the "heart failure" response in these patients is therefore very different to that seen in non-congenital disease, albeit with an almost identical phenotype. Furthermore, it would be predicted from this data that these patients would be unlikely to respond to classical heart

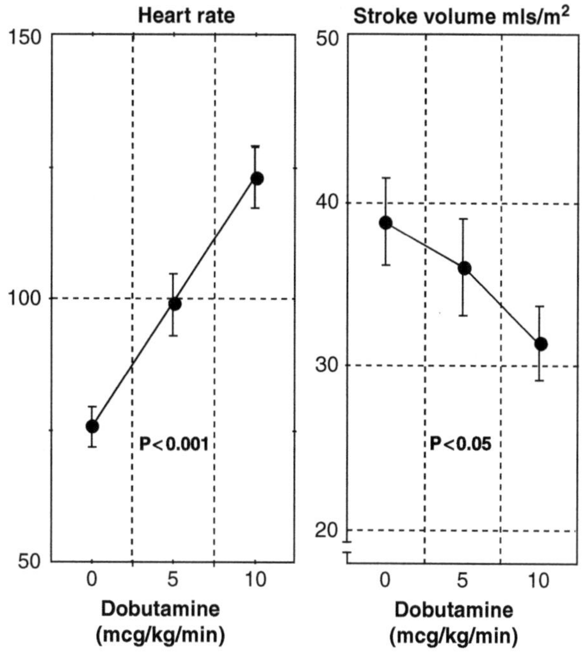

Fig. 6.3 Datare drawnfr om Derrick et al.[32] (see text for details). In patients after Mustard and Senning procedures, an increase in heart rate (*left panel*)d uring dobutamine infusion is associated with a fall in stroke volume (*right panel*). The mechanism for this is a fixed ventricular filling rate due to non-capacitant atrial baffles, not "right ventricular failure"

failure treatment. Indeed, these patients seem resistant to the effect of angiotensin converting enzyme inhibition and angiotensin receptor blockade,[33] the latter being studied in a randomized, double-blind, placebo-controlled trial showing no benefit from these drugs in terms of right ventricular functional performance or exercise abilities.

The right ventricle in congenitally corrected transposition (CCTGA) might be considered a purer form of systemic right ventricle. Even in the absence of previous surgical intervention and without significant associated abnormalities, the functional decline in these patients is well known.[34] Again, we must ask ourselves what is the evidence for an intrinsic right ventricular myocardial problem under these circumstances? While there are case reports describing survival of undiagnosed cases into late old age,[35] this cannot be used as convincing evidence for the lack of an intrinsic myocardial problem. However, there is more robust data to support the notion that myocardial failure is not the entire problem. For example, in a study describing the outcome of a large group of patients with congenitally corrected transposition, it was shown that long term symptom free survival was, as expected, markedly abnormal compared to the normal population.[36] However, when those patients with only trivial or mild tricuspid incompetence were compared with those with moderate and severe tricuspid incompetence, there was a very marked difference. Those with trivial or mild tricuspid incompetence having virtually normal symptom free survival.[36]

While for some, tricuspid incompetence is intrinsic to the disease (those with Ebstein's anomaly of the tricuspid valve for example) for many this is a progressive and acquired lesion. Again, we can look to biventricular interactions as the fundamental basis for this pathophysiology. As discussed earlier, the tricuspid valve is characterized by the insertion of its subvalve apparatus into the septal surface. In CCTGA the left ventricle does not assume its normal prolate ellipsoid shape, the result being that the septum becomes convex toward the right ventricle. Further septal shift can further displace the tricuspid valve septal leaflet away from its counterparts setting up a vicious cycle of right heart dilatation begetting worse tricuspid regurgitation.[37] While tricuspid valve replacement is a viable alternative for many,[38] the results of this strategy have been variable from institution to institution.[39] An understanding of the fundamental pathophysiology, allows potential alternative strategies for the treatment of these patients. The use of pulmonary artery banding, to reverse this septal shift and restore tricuspid valve competency is now widely reported.[40] Again, it is beyond the scope of this chapter to discuss the literature in detail, but suffice it to say that there are many caviats and dogmas associated with such therapy. Pulmonary artery banding to "retrain" the subpulmonary left ventricle is thought to be limited to the young child and early adolescence.[41] Indeed many authors have advised against such therapy in older adolescents and adults.[40] While it is clear that the latter group have less satisfactory outcomes, this may be more a result of imperfect banding procedures than an intrinsic inability to retrain the more aged left ventricle. Indeed, it appears that the induction of left ventricular dysfunction during pulmonary artery banding, no matter when it is performed, is the most important factor in failure of this strategy, rather than age per se.[41] We clearly have much to learn about the optimal methods of retraining. Nonetheless, pulmonary artery banding with a view to a double switch type procedure, or maybe even as destination therapy, is an intriguing form of harnessing these potentially adverse biventricular interactions for clinical benefit. Again, there clearly will be more research needed before specific guidelines and outlines can be defined.

6.5.4 The Right Ventricle in the Functionally Univentricular Circulation

Finally we should discuss the situation where the right ventricle is the only functional, or dominant, ventricle within the circulation. While clearly "biventricular" interactions are less overt, there remains substantial concern regarding the long term viability of these ventricles in such circulations.

Numerically, the commonest form of functionally single right ventricle is the hypoplastic left heart syndrome. The first question to ask, in terms of the right ventricle being able to perform adequately within this circulation, is whether hypoplastic left heart syndrome itself is a risk factor for early outcomes of staged palliation? Interestingly, there is remarkably little data relating right ventricular dysfunction to the outcomes of the initial Norwood procedure. In one study, poor right ventricular ejection fraction was not associated with reduced early survival, but appeared to predict worse outcomes at 12–24 months.[42] In more recent studies, right ventricular ejection fraction has emerged as a stronger predictor of outcomes of the Norwood procedure.[43] Nonetheless, if the right ventricle were intrinsically a "weaker" ventricle, then one might expect hypoplastic left heart syndrome to be a risk factor for poorer outcomes after the Fontan procedure. In this regard, the data are beginning to suggest a difference between short and medium term outcomes and the longer term outcomes. Two studies have failed to show a disadvantage from having a systemic right ventricle in the

Fontan circulation. The Children's Hospital of Philadelphia asked the question as to whether hypoplastic left heart syndrome was a risk factor for the Fontan procedure.[44] The answer from their data was a resounding no. Similarly, an analysis of the outcomes of Fontan procedures at Boston Children's Hospital showed that those with a functionally single right ventricle, or those with a functionally single left ventricle and normally related great arteries, fared better than all other patients in terms of Kaplan Meier survival.[45] Nonetheless, there are emerging data from large cross sectional data sets suggesting that the right ventricle is disadvantaged in the long-term. The Pediatric Heart Network have produced important data in this regard. Analyzing the data from over 500 patients across multiple institutions, the presence of a systemic right ventricle did appear to predict worse exercise performance.[46] In addition, abnormalities of systolic and diastolic function were more prevalent in those with a systemic right ventricle in another study.[47] However, the direct consequences, in terms of symptoms and long term outcomes, remain to be defined.

Clearly chronic therapies to reduce the incidence of functional decline would be advantageous in this group of patients whether they have a functionally single left or right ventricle. Unfortunately, as with most areas of congenital heart disease, those therapies well defined for the treatment of adult acquired heart failure have proven unsuccessful in the treatment of the staged Fontan. In a Pediatric Heart Network study recently presented in abstract form, angiotensin converting enzyme inhibition failed to impact ventricular performance or growth prior to the bidirectional Glenn procedure. In another randomized double blind placebo controlled trial of, albeit a small number, of post-Fontan patients, ACE inhibition had no effect on functional performance, and perhaps even worsened exercise related stroke volume responses in the treatment group.[48] The effects of beta blockade have been similarly disappointing. In fact, the effects of beta blockade may be adverse to the failing subpulmonary or systemic right ventricle. In the Carvedilol trial described in detail elsewhere, those with ventricular morphology other than a left ventricle appeared to be worse during treatment, than with placebo.[49]

6.6 Summary and Conclusion

We can no longer ignore the role of the right ventricle in heart failure syndromes, even when normally situated in its subpulmonary position, and relatively unaffected directly by the disease at hand. In congenital heart diseases, symptoms and outcome may be driven primarily by abnormalities of right ventricular form and function. As the importance of right ventricular dysfunction has emerged, the importance of biventricular interactions has become better understood, even in conditions considered to be associated with "isolated" right or left ventricular dysfunction. For the time being, our ability to modify these diseases relies on mechanical or electromechanical interventions. Pharmacologic support of the failing right ventricle has been almost uniformly unsuccessful to date. Hopefully with better understanding of the mechanisms of functional decline in association with right ventricular dysfunction, our ability to prevent and treat the increasing number of patients with the potential for right ventricular failure will improve in the future.

References

1. Zornoff LA, Skali H, Pfeffer MA, St John Sutton M, Rouleau JL, Lamas GA, Plappert T, Rouleau JR, Moyé LA, Lewis SJ, Braunwald E, Solomon SD; SAVE Investigators. Right ventricular dysfunction and risk of heart failure and mortality after myocardial infarction. *J Am Coll Cardiol.* May 1, 2002;39(9):1450–1455.
2. Srivastava D. Making or breaking the heart: from lineage determination to morphogenesis. *Cell.*2006;126:1 037–1048.
3. Mori AD, Zhu Y, Vahora I, Nieman B, Koshiba-Takeuchi K, Davidson L, Pizard A, Seidman JG, Seidman CE, Chen XJ, Henkelman RM, Bruneau BG. Tbx5-dependent rheostatic control of cardiac gene expression and morphogenesis. *Dev Biol.* September 15, 2006;297(2):566–586.
4. Rouleau JL, Paradis P, Shenasa H, Juneau C. Faster time to peak tension and velocity of shortening in right versus left ventricular trabeculae and papillary muscles of dogs. *Circ Res.* November1986; 59(5):556–561.
5. Anderson RH, Ho SY. What is a ventricle? *Ann Thorac Surg.*A ugust1998; 66(2):616–620.
6. Merrick AF, Yacoub MH, Ho SY, Anderson RH. Anatomy of the muscular subpulmonary infundibulum with regard to the Ross procedure. *Ann Thorac Surg.* February 2006;69(2): 556–561.
7. Torrent-Guasp F. La estructuracion macroscopica del miocardio ventricular rev esp cardiol 1980;33265–33287.
8. LeGrice IJ. et al. Laminar structure of the heart: ventricular myocyte arrangement and connective tissue architectue in the dog. *Am J Physiol.* 1995;269(2 pt 2):H571–H582.
9. Sanchez-Quintana D et al. Myoarchitecture and connective tissue in hearts with tricuspid atresia. *Heart.*1999; 81:182–191.
10. Redington A. et al. Characterisation of the normal right ventricular pressure volume relation by biplane angiography an simultaneous micromanometer pressure measurements. i. 1988;59:23–30.
11. Shaver JA. Clinical implications of the hangout interval. *Int J Cardiolo.* March 1984;5(3): 391–398.
12. Suga H, Sagawa K, Shoukas A. Load independence of the instantaneous Pressure-Volume Ratio of the Canine Left Ventricle and effects of Epinephrine and heart rate on the Ratio Circ Res.1973:314–3 22.
13. Konstantinov IE, Saxena P, Koniuszko MD, Alvarez J, Newman MA. Acute massive pulmonary embolism with cardiopulmonary resuscitation: management and results. *Tex Heart Inst J.* 2007;34(1):41–45.
14. Damiano J. Significant left ventricular contribution to right ventricular systolic function. *Am J Physiol Heart Circ Physiol.*1991; 261:H1514–H1524.
15. Hoffman D. Left-to-right ventricular interaction with a non contracting right ventricle. *J Thorac Cardiovasc Surg.*1994; 107:1496–1502.
16. Brookes C. et al. Acute right ventricular dilatation in response to Ischemia significantly impairs left ventricular systolic performance. *Circulation.*1999; 100:761–767.
17. Redington AN et al. Changes in the pressure-volume relation of the right ventricle when its loading conditions are modified. *Br Heart J.*J anuary1990; 63(1):45–49.
18. Gaynor SL, Maniar HS, Bloch JB, Steendijk P, Moon MR. Right atrial and ventricular adaptation to chronic right ventricular pressure overload. *Circulation.* August 30, 2005; 112(9s uppl):I212–218.
19. Hopkins WE. The remarkable right ventricle of patients with Eisenmenger syndrome. *Coron Artery Dis.*Fe bruary2005; 16(1):19–25.
20. Stojnic BB, Brecker SJ, Xiao HB, Helmy SM, Mbaissouroum M, Gibson DG. Left ventricular filling characteristics in pulmonary hypertension: a new mode of ventricular interaction. *Br Heart J.*J uly 1992;68(1):16–20.

21. Curtiss EI, Reddy PS, O'Toole JD, Shaver JA. Alterations of right ventricular systolic time intervals by chronic pressure and volume overloading. *Circulation.* June 1976;53(6): 997–1003.
22. Gan CT, Lankhaar JW, Marcus JT, Westerhof N, Marques KM, Bronzwaer JG, Boonstra A, Postmus PE, Vonk-Noordegraaf A. Impaired left ventricular filling due to right-to-left ventricular interaction in patients with pulmonary arterial hypertension. *Am J Physiol Heart Circ Physiol.*A pril2006; 290(4):H1528–H1533.
23. Alkon J, Humpl T, Manlhiot C, McCrindle BW, Reyes J, Friedberg M. The right ventricular S:D ratio is significant predictor of outcomes in children with pulmonary arterial hypertension. *J Am Soc Echocardiograph.*2009; 22:551–552.
24. Holverda S, Gan CT, Marcus JT, Postmus PE, Boonstra A, Vonk-Noordegraaf A. Impaired stroke volume response to exercise in pulmonary arterial hypertension. *J Am Coll Cardiol.* April 18, 2006;47(8):1732–1733.
25. Labombarda F, Maragnes P, Dupont-Chauvet P, Serraf A. Potts anastomosis for children with idiopathic pulmonary hypertension. *Pediatr Cardiol.*N ovember2009; 30(8):1143–1145.
26. Apitz C, Webb GD, Redington AN. Tetralogy of Fallot. *Lancet.* October 24, 2009; 374(9699):1462–1471.
27. Davlouros PA, Kilner PJ, Hornung TS, Li W, Francis JM, Moon JC, Smith GC, Tat T, Pennell DJ, Gatzoulis MA. Right ventricular function in adults with repaired tetralogy of Fallot assessed with cardiovascular magnetic resonance imaging: detrimental role of right ventricular outflow aneurysms or akinesia and adverse right-to-left ventricular interaction. *J Am Coll Cardiol.* December 4, 2002;40(11):2044–2052.
28. Ghai A, Silversides C, Harris L, Webb GD, Siu SC, Therrien J. Left ventricular dysfunction is a risk factor for sudden cardiac death in adults late after repair of tetralogy of Fallot. *J Am Coll Cardiol.* November 6, 2002;40(9):1675–1680.
29. Tobler D, Crean A, Oechslin E, Silversides C, Wald R, Redington A, Van Arsdell G, Caldarone C. Left Ventricular Function After Pulmonary Valve Replacement in Adults After Repair of Tetralogy of Fallot. Abstract presented 2009 Scientific Sessions of American Heart Association.
30. D'Andrea A, Caso P, Sarubbi B, D'Alto M, Giovanna Russo M, Scherillo M, Cotrufo M, Calabrò R. Right ventricular myocardial activation delay in adult patients with right bundle branch block late after repair of Tetralogy of Fallot. *Eur J Echocardiogr.* March 2004;5(2): 123–131.
31. Kirsh JA, Stephenson EA, Redington AN. Images in cardiovascular medicine. Recovery of left ventricular systolic function after biventricular resynchronization pacing in a child with repaired tetralogy of Fallot and severe biventricular dysfunction. *Circulation.* April 11, 2006;113(14):e691–e692.
32. Derrick GP, Narang I, White PA, Kelleher A, Bush A, Penny DJ, Redington AN. Failure of stroke volume augmentation during exercise and dobutamine stress is unrelated to load-independent indexes of right ventricular performance after the Mustard operation. *Circulation.* November 7, 2007;102(19 suppl 3):III154–III159.
33. Dore A, Houde C, Chan KL, Ducharme A, Khairy P, Juneau M, Marcotte F, Mercier LA. Angiotensin receptor blockade and exercise capacity in adults with systemic right ventricles: a multicenter, randomized, placebo-controlled clinical trial. *Circulation.* October 18, 2005;112(16):2411–2416.
34. Graham TP Jr. et al. Long-term outcome in congenitally corrected transposition of the great arteries: a multi-intitutional study. *J Am Coll Cardiol.*20 00;36(1):255–261.
35. Roffi M, de Marchi SF, Seiler C. Congenitally corrected transposition of the great arteries in an 80 year old woman. *Heart.*J une1998; 79(6):622–623.
36. Prieto L et al. Progressive tricuspid valve disease in patients with congenitally corrected transposition of the great arteries. *Circulation.*1998; 98(10):997–1005.

37. Jahangiri M, Redington AN, Elliott MJ, Stark J, Tsang VT, de Leval MR. A case for anatomic correction in atrioventricular discordance? Effects of surgery on tricuspid valve function. *J Thorac Cardiovasc Surg*.J une2001; 121(6):1040–1045.
38. van Son JA, Danielson GK, Huhta JC, Warnes CA, Edwards WD, Schaff HV, Puga FJ, Ilstrup DM. Late results of systemic atrioventricular valve replacement in corrected transposition. *J Thorac Cardiovasc Surg*.A pril1995; 109(4):642–652.
39. Hraska V, Duncan BW, Mayer JE Jr, Freed M, del Nido PJ, Jonas RA. Long-term outcome of surgically treated patients with corrected transposition of the great arteries. *J Thorac Cardiovasc Surg*.J anuary2005; 129(1):182–191.
40. Winlaw DS, McGuirk SP, Balmer C, Langley SM, Griselli M, Stümper O, De Giovanni JV, right JG, Thorne S, Barron DJ, Brawn WJ. Intention-to-treat analysis of pulmonary artery banding in conditions with a morphological right ventricle in the systemic circulation with a view to anatomic biventricular repair. *Circulation*. February 1, 2005;111(4):405–411.
41. Mee RB. The double switch operation with accent on the Senning component. *Semin Thorac Cardiovasc Surg Pediatr Card Surg Annu*.2005: 57–65.
42. Altmann K, Printz BF, Solowiejczky DE, Gersony WM, Quaegebeur J, Apfel HD. Two-dimensional echocardiographic assessment of right ventricular function as a predictor of outcome in hypoplastic left heart syndrome. *Am J Cardiol*. November 1, 2000;86(9):964–968.
43. Walsh MA, McCrindle BW, Dipchand A, Manlhiot C, Hickey E, Caldarone CA, Van Arsdell GS, Schwartz SM. Left ventricular morphology influences mortality after the Norwood operation. *Heart*.A ugust2009; 95(15):1238–1244.
44. Gaynor JW, Bridges ND, Cohen MI, Mahle WT, Decampli WM, Steven JM, Nicolson SC, Spray TL. Predictors of outcome after the Fontan operation: is hypoplastic left heart syndrome still a risk factor? *J Thorac Cardiovasc Surg*.Fe bruary2002; 123(2):237–245.
45. Gentles TL, Mayer JE Jr, Gauvreau K, Newburger JW, Lock JE, Kupferschmid JP, Burnett J, Jonas RA, Castañeda AR, Wernovsky G. Fontan operation in five hundred consecutive patients: factors influencing early and late outcome. *J Thorac Cardiovasc Surg*. September 1997;114(3):376–391.
46. Paridon SM, Mitchell PD, Colan SD, Williams RV, Blaufox A, Li JS, Margossian R, Mital S, Russell J, Rhodes J; Pediatric Heart Network Investigators. Across-sectional study of exercise performance during the first 2 decades of life after the Fontan operation. *J Am Coll Cardiol*. July 8, 2008;52(2):99–107.
47. Anderson PA, Sleeper LA, Mahony L, Colan SD, Atz AM, Breitbart RE, Gersony WM, Gallagher D, Geva T, Margossian R, McCrindle BW, Paridon S, Schwartz M, Stylianou M, Williams RV, Clark BJ 3rd; Pediatric Heart Network Investigators. Contemporary outcomes after the Fontan procedure: a Pediatric Heart Network multicenter study. *J Am Coll Cardiol*. July 8, 2008;52(2):85–98.
48. Kouatli AA, Garcia JA, Zellers TM, Weinstein EM, Mahony L. Enalapril does not enhance exercise capacity in patients after Fontan procedure. *Circulation*. September 2, 1997;96(5): 1507–1512.
49. Shaddy RE, Boucek MM, Hsu DT, Boucek RJ, Canter CE, Mahony L, Ross RD, Pahl E, Blume ED, Dodd DA, Rosenthal DN, Burr J, LaSalle B, Holubkov R, Lukas MA, Tani LY; Pediatric Carvedilol Study Group. Carvedilol for children and adolescents with heart failure: a randomized controlled trial. *JAMA*.Se ptember12,2007; 298(10):1171–1179.

Mechanical Circulatory Support in the Patientwi th Congenital Heart Disease

7

Chitra Ravishankar, Troy E. Dominguez, Tami M. Rosenthal, and J. William Gaynor

7.1 History and Introduction

While conventional therapy with inotropic support and afterload reduction remains the mainstay of treatment for the failing heart, mechanical circulatory support is being increasingly used in the pediatric population.[1–5] The majority of the pediatric experience consists of use of extracorporeal membrane oxygenation (ECMO). ECMO which is the use of mechanical devices to replace heart and lung function for cardiopulmonary failure was first used successfully for cardiac failure in a child in 1972, and respiratory failure in a neonate in 1975. In September 2004, the Extracorporeal Life Support Organization (ELSO) celebrated its 15th anniversary by honoring Dr. Robert Bartlett, the founding father of ECMO. A young woman called Esperanza was also present as an invited guest; she was the first survivor of ECMO. Esperanza which means "hope" in Spanish was an abandoned newborn with respiratory failure who was failing conventional therapy. Dr. Bartlett and his colleagues were working in the laboratory on modification of the cardiopulmonary bypass circuit for use in respiratory failure in children. When consulted about this sick neonate, they decided to utilize their laboratory experience in a clinical setting as a "bench to bedside" effort[6]. The rest as they say is history. The success of ECMO in neonates with respiratory failure led to wider application to treatment of cardiac failure as a bridge to recovery or transplantation, and as a bridge to a long-term ventricular assist device (VAD) in the current era. ELSO was established in 1989 to share experience, education, and to maintain a registry of cases[7]. There are now more than 40,000 patents in the registry including over 9,000 pediatric cardiac cases.

Long-term VAD support as a bridge to transplantation has been available for treatment of heart failure in adults for over two decades. Adult devices have been successfully used in older children and adolescents; however these devices are not suitable for use in neonates, infants and young children. Thus mechanical circulatory support in

C. Ravishankar (✉)
Department of Pediatrics, The Children's Hospital of Philadelphia Civic Center Boulevard
Philadelphia,P A19 104-4399,U SA
e-mail:ra vishankar@email.chop.edu

R.E. Shaddy (ed.), *Heart Failure in Congenital Heart Disease*,
DOI: 10.1007/978-1-84996-480-7_7, © Springer-Verlag London Limited 2011

children was limited to short-term support with ECMO, or the ECMO circuit without an oxygenator using a centrifugal pump. An infant was supported for the first time with a paracorporeal pneumatic device using a 10 mL pump (Berlin Heart EXCOR) in Germany in 1992. This device was approved by the Food and Drug Administration (FDA) for compassionate use in the United States in 2004, and there is an ongoing trial in North America to evaluate the safety and efficacy of this device. Thus with the advent of new technology, long-term ventricular assist devices (VAD) are being increasingly used in infants, children and young adults as a bridge to transplantation.[8–10] The majority of the VAD experience is in children with cardiomyopathy. Children with congenital heart disease (CHD) present unique challenges due to complex anatomy and physiology (including but not limited to patients with single ventricle physiology), presence of hypoxemia, and pulmonary hypertension.

In this chapter, we review the types of mechanical circulatory support (Table 7.1), indications for ECMO, the currently available systems, and the pediatric experience with the use of ECMO and VAD, mechanical circulatory support in children with single ventricle physiology, and emerging new technology. This review will focus on mechanical circulatory support in children with CHD.

7.2 Types of Mechanical Circulatory Support

Table 7.1 summarizes the available devices in children categorized by the anticipated duration of support. ECMO, centrifugal pumps, and the long-term devices will be further explored in this chapter. A comparison of ECMO versus VAD is provided later in the chapter(seeT able 7.4).

Table7. 1 Typesofme chanicalc irculatorys upport

Short-term (days to weeks)
ECMO
Intra-aortic balloon counterpulsation
Bio-pump (centrifugal pump)
Abiomed BVS 5000
Long-termde vices
Thoratec (pulsatile, paracorporeal, pneumatic)
Heartmate LVAS (pulsatile, implantable, electric)
Berlin Heart EXCOR (pulsatile, paracorporeal, pneumatic)
Medos HIA-VAD (pulsatile, paracorporeal, pneumatic)
DeBakey VAD Child (axial, implantable, electric)

Modified from Blume ED, Laussen PC. Cardiac Mechanical Support Therapies. Moss And Adams' Heart Disease in Infants, Children, and Adolescents, 7th edition, 2008

7.3 Indications for Mechanical Circulatory Support

7.3.1 Pre-operativeS tabilization

Mechanical circulatory support is occasionally required in neonates who present with airway obstruction, profound cyanosis and/or cardiogenic shock (Table 7.2). Examples include patients with obstructed total anomalous pulmonary venous connection, and tetralogy of Fallot with absent pulmonary valve syndrome who may present in extremis. Preoperative stabilization with ECMO support provides time for organ recovery and diagnostic testing prior to surgery. Pulmonary hypertension refractory to conventional therapy can occur in neonates with transposition of great arteries and there are several reports of the successful use of ECMO for pre-operative stabilization.[11] ECMO can also be beneficial in infants with arrhythmias refractory to medical therapy (e.g. severe Ebstein's anomaly of the tricuspid valve with supraventricular tachycardia), or for pre-operative stabilization in neonates with respiratory failure from severe tracheal stenosis (e.g. left pulmonary artery sling with tracheal rings).[12,13] Another example is the neonate with severe Ebstein's anomaly and functional pulmonary atresia with ductal-dependant pulmonary blood flow, who has a circular shunt from a wide open ductus arteriosus, and will benefit from ECMO support while the pulmonary vascular resistance declines.[14]

7.3.2 Post-cardiotomy Cardio-Pulmonary Insufficiency

This is the most common indication for mechanical circulatory support in children with CHD as a bridge to recovery or transplantation. ECMO may be required in the postoperative period either due to the inability to separate from cardiopulmonary bypass (CPB), progressive low cardiac output syndrome (LCOS), or cardiac arrest caused by a number of factors such as ventricular dysfunction, pulmonary hypertension, progressive hypoxemia or intractable arrhythmias. Risk factors include prolonged cardiopulmonary bypass (CPB) time and aortic cross clamp time, pre-existing ventricular dysfunction (e.g. anomalous left coronary artery from pulmonary artery or ALCAPA), or the acute

Table7. 2 Indications

Preoperatives tabilization
Post-cardiotomys upport
E-CPR (ecmo for cardiopulmonary resuscitation)
Bridge to cardiac transplantation

change in loading condition that occurs with relief of long-standing atrioventricular valve regurgitation.[15] The majority of patients requiring ECMO immediately after CPB remain cannulated via the median sternotomy with an atrial cannula for venous drainage and an arterial cannula in the aorta. Patients requiring ECMO in the intensive care unit are more likely to be cannulated via the right internal jugular vein and right carotid artery. Decompression of the ventricle with a left atrial vent is often needed to prevent ventricular distention (which impedes recovery) and left atrial hypertension (which may cause pulmonary hemorrhage). Hemorrhage is a major complication of ECMO after cardiac surgery, and mediastinal exploration is often necessary with transthoracic cannulation.

Due consideration should be given to placing a patient on ECMO 'urgently" in the intensive care unit for progressive LCOS before the onset of irreversible organ dysfunction, rather than 'emergently" during a cardiac arrest. Irrespective of timing of ECMO cannulation, it is important to rule out significant residual lesions using echocardiography and cardiac catheterization if necessary, especially if myocardial recovery does not occur as anticipated, and the patient fails to wean off the ECMO circuit within 48–72 h. This will also help clinicians make a decision about listing for heart transplantation if end organ function is preserved or restored, and/or placement of a long-term VAD.

7.3.4 ECMO for Resuscitation During Cardiopulmonary Arrest or E-CPR

Del Nido et al. initially described the use of rapid resuscitation ECMO after cardiopulmonary arrest (CPR). Many centers now have the capability of rapid deployment of ECMO and current survival for this indication is 40–50%.[16–18] Rapid institution of circulatory support with modified ECMO systems can be lifesaving with better preservation of end-organ function in these patients. A rapid deployment team usually includes a cardiac intensivist, cardiac surgeon, cardiology fellow, perfusionist or ECMO technician, a scrub nurse, cardiac anesthesiologist, and a senior cardiac nurse. ECMO should be considered for patients who have suffered a witnessed arrest with rapid institution of CPR and no recovery of cardiac function within 5–10 min of the event. Once this decision has been made, an attempt should be made to maintain adequate blood pressure with chest compressions rather than pharmacologic therapy with vasoconstrictors such as epinephrine. Topical hypothermia with application of ice to the head is also advocated during resuscitation. Determination of eligibility for E-CPR during active resuscitation is obviously challenging. In general children with biventricular circulation and single ventricle patients with a shunt dependant circulation are candidates for E-CPR in the absence of major co-morbidities. On the other hand, children with cavopulmonary connections are not good candidates for E-CPR as they are at risk of sustaining significant neurologic damage during resuscitation due to cerebral venous hypertension. Besides, ECMO can be technically quite challenging with cavopulmonary connections (see section on single ventricle patients).

7.3.5 Bridge to Heart Transplantation

Long-term VADs are being increasingly used in children for this indication.[9,19] A majority of this experience is in children with dilated cardiomyopathy. With the advent of new technology, pulsatile devices are available for use in infants (Berlin heart and Medos), and older children (Thoratec, Heartmate, Abiomed). VAD support should be anticipated and every attempt must be made to initiate VAD support "urgently" rather than "emergently" before the onset of irreversible end organ dysfunction or circulatory collapse. If necessary, support with ECMO can be utilized as a bridge to longer term VAD. Similar to children with end stage heart failure in the setting of dilated cardiomyopathy, feeding intolerance or abdominal pain and loss of appetite are ominous symptoms in children with CHD. If these symptoms do not respond to escalation of inotropic support and afterload reduction, VAD support should be considered. Unlike children with cardiomyopathy, a majority of children with CHD have a history of prior sternotomy and/or cardiac catheterization. Femoral vessels and neck vessels should be screened for patency using ultrasonography, both to determine sites for emergent cannulation for ECMO or an alternate site for cannulation for CPB during placement of VAD.

In the current era, ECMO in children with biventricular circulation is viewed as a short-term bridge to heart transplantation due to the attendant risks associated with ECMO and prolonged waiting time for heart transplantation. For any given patient on ECMO, in the absence of residual lesions amenable to surgery, and with inadequate myocardial recovery to safely wean off ECMO support within 48–72 h, serious consideration should be given to transitioning from ECMO to a long-term VAD.

7.4 ECMO

The need for ECMO in neonatal respiratory failure has declined as a result of newer therapies such as surfactant, inspired nitric oxide, and high frequency oscillatory ventilation. As opposed to the use of ECMO in neonatal respiratory failure, the use of ECMO for pediatric cardiac failure has been increasing with time. Unlike ECMO for respiratory indications, venoarterial or VA ECMO is used for cardiac indications since circulatory support is usually required. The rest of this review will pertain to VA ECMO.

7.4.1 The Circuit

The ECMO circuit is complex with cannulae, tubing, multiple monitors, flow meters, and ports. However, there are three main components of the ECMO circuit:

1. Apum p
2. Am embraneoxyge nator
3. Ahe ate xchanger

Venous drainage occurs by gravity to the pump and negative pressure created by the pump head. With the most common type of pump, a roller pump, servo-regulation occurs using a venous reservoir. If excessive negative pressures are detected in the reservoir, the pump stops to prevent gas embolization, through "cavitation" of gas out of the blood phase, and hemolysis. The roller pump consists of a rotating roller head that compresses blood through a section of tubing lying within a circular plate. Some centers prefer the use of a centrifugal pump which is a device that generates flow from a spinning rotor that draws blood in centrally from the venous cannula that is then displaced centrifugally outward through an opening in the device directly to the membrane oxygenator or arterial cannula. The Better-Bladder (BB) is a new online device that is used in many centers in the United States. The BB is a length of standard perfusion tubing with a thin walled, sausage shaped balloon sealed within a clear, rigid housing. It provides compliance in the venous line and allows for noninvasive pressure measurements. Both features are useful for controlling pump speed as a function of venous line pressure.

From the pump, blood travels to the membrane oxygenator where gas exchange occurs. Two types of oxygenators are in common use: *silicone membrane oxygenators* and *hollow-fiber oxygenators*. Sweep gas is delivered into the gas inlet of the membrane oxygenator so that O_2 and CO_2 can be transferred across the membrane into the blood and gas phases. The excess gas flow then exits the gas outlet port. Gas exchange is dependent upon the oxygenator diffusion characteristics, surface area, blood film thickness, blood flow rate, gas concentration gradients, and sweep gas flow. The sweep gas flow rate regulates CO_2 elimination and the oxygen blender regulates the delivered oxygen, and thus the oxygen content of blood leaving the membrane oxygenator. Sweep gas flow rate does not affect O_2 delivery; the F_iO_2 of the sweep gas changes O_2 delivery. The surface area of oxygenator limits the maximum rates of blood flow and sweep gas flow through the oxygenator, and therefore gas exchange. More recently, a diffusion membrane (Quadrox) has been used by many centers especially in Europe. The miniaturized version, "Quadrox-I" has recently been approved by the FDA. This device provides efficient gas transfer with a low pressure drop.

Heat loss occurs from extracorporeal circulation making a heat exchanger necessary to regulate body temperature. The blood is warmed by a water-jacketed heat exchanger that is incorporated into the oxygenator design or by a separate heat exchanger after leaving the membrane oxygenator prior to entering the patient. An overall schematic for a general ECMO circuit containing the above components is given in Fig. 7.1.

For VA ECMO, cannulation is usually performed via transthoracic or transcervical approach. The former involves placement of the venous drainage cannula into the jugular vein to drain the right atrium. The arterial cannula is then placed into carotid artery with the tip in the ascending aorta. Transthoracic cannulation is frequently utilized in postoperative cardiac patients. In this instance, the right atrium is drained by direct cannulation and there is arterial return by direct cannulation of the ascending aorta. Select patients may benefit from VA ECMO via the femoral approach. However, this type of support could be

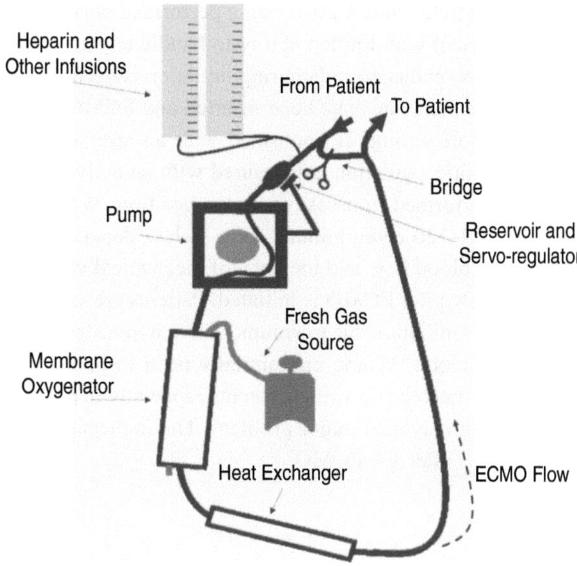

Fig. 7.1 Schematic for a general ECMO circuit

problematic if there is significant lung injury since it is possible for desaturated blood from the left ventricle to perfuse the coronaries, head, and neck vessels and impair oxygen delivery to these vital organs. There is also an increased risk of leg ischemia with cannulation of the femoral vessel, and this approach is unsuitable for small infants due to the small size of the vessels.

7.4.2 Management

7.4.2.1 Initiation

The decision to place a patient on ECMO is often an emergent or urgent situation in the setting of circulatory failure. ECMO can either be used as a bridge to recovery if the etiology of the cardio- respiratory failure is reversible or as a bridge to heart transplantation or long-term ventricular assist device in the absence of recovery of myocardial function. Most commonly, vascular access is obtained by the surgical team, but there may be some circumstances where access is obtained percutaneously by the intensive care team. The intensive care team should discuss the access sites to be prepared and positioning of the patient with the surgeon. A dose of unfractionated heparin (50–100 units per kilogram) is made available and given prior to cannulation at the discretion of the surgeon. The ECMO specialist or perfusionist builds and prepares the circuit concomitantly or acquires a pre-primed circuit. Additional blood prime will be necessary in smaller patients due to hemodilution. With E-CPR, an individual or two will need to be sterile so as not to contaminate the surgical field while CPR is being performed during cannulation. The ECMO circuit is a closed circuit with limited ability to handle any air in the venous limb, and careful de-airing of the venous cannula during initiation is necessary.

After the cannulae have been inserted and ECMO flow increased, the adequacy of the initial support settings is confirmed with an arterial blood gas and hemodynamics, the degree of anticoagulation is measured with an activated clotting time, and a chest radiograph is performed to assess cannulae position. When VA ECMO is performed at flow rates of 100–120 cc/kg/minute, there is less dependence of gas exchange on antegrade pulmonary blood flow and the level of mechanical ventilation can be reduced to "rest settings" shortly after ECMO is initiated. Patients are vulnerable to hemodynamic instability with ECMO initiation due to volume shifts, hypocalcemia, or electrolyte disturbances. The circulating blood volume may initially need to be augmented with crystalloid or blood products to meet the flow requirements especially in post-cardiotomy patients where ongoing bleeding may be a major problem. The inotropic support can also usually be rapidly discontinued after VA ECMO.

7.4.2.2 Left Ventricular Decompression

To maximize the chance for myocardial recovery, it is important to reduce the wall stress of the ventricle and maximize myocardial oxygen delivery. With severely compromised ventricular function, the systemic ventricle may be unable to eject the volume of blood returned to it via antegrade pulmonary blood flow, thebesian veins, and bronchial blood flow. When this happens, the resultant ventricular distension and elevated end-diastolic pressure can lead to increase in wall stress, impaired coronary perfusion, and irreversible myocardial ischemia. Additionally, the elevated left ventricular end-diastolic pressure can result in pulmonary venous hypertension, pulmonary edema, and pulmonary hemorrhage. Left atrial decompression either through balloon atrial septostomy or venting of the left atrium can reverse this physiology, improve the pulmonary status, and optimize the chance for ventricular recovery.[20] Flow rates of 100–150 cc/kg/min should allow good systemic oxygen delivery and unloading of the ventricle to allow recovery of ventricular function. Afterload reducing agents such as milrinone may also be necessary.

7.4.2.3 Ventilation

Most patients requiring cardiac ECMO do not have significant pulmonary dysfunction. Therefore, lung protective strategies are less important in this population. Additionally, the levels of positive end-expiratory pressure necessary are generally $\leq$5 cm H_2O. A minimal tidal volume is utilized to prevent atelactasis. Ventilator rates are usually minimized since CO_2 elimination is frequently quite efficient using the membrane oxygenator. In fact, it may be necessary to blend CO_2 with the sweep gas in order to normalize the arterial pCO_2.

7.4.2.4 Sedation

Neuromuscular blockade is rarely necessary except during cannulation or decannulation. The dosages of some drugs may need to be increased due to absorption by the circuit, additional blood volume from the circuit for drug distribution, or increased drug clearance with the use of hemofiltration. For example, fentanyl has been shown to irreversibly bind to the membrane oxygenator and circuit, but may saturate the circuit with long term use. Both fentanyl and morphine requirements have been reported to increased on ECMO. Given this unpredictability, it is most prudent to titrate sedative and analgesic drugs to effect. Since a patient's neurologic status is frequently of concern while on ECMO, it is often best to minimize the use of heavy sedation. Inhaled anesthetic gas (isoflurane) may be blended in with the sweep gas to provide sedation, afterload reduction, and allow neurologic function to be assessed fairly rapidly once discontinued.

Given the potential gravity of neurologic complications in ECMO patients, screening head ultrasonography is performed in infants and frequent neurologic assessment is performed in all age groups. In older pediatric patients, a head computed tomography scan may be necessary to define the extent of the neurologic insult. In treating seizures, larger loading and maintenance doses of anti-seizure medications may be necessary to obtain optimal serum concentrations. In addition, drug re-dosing may be needed with circuit changes.

7.4.2.5 Fluids/Nutrition

Systemic inflammation and capillary leak may occur after initiating ECMO. Intravenous fluid volume is usually minimized and diuretics are frequently given in the form of bolus or continuous infusion. Enteral feedings have been shown to be cost-effective and well tolerated while pediatric patients are on ECMO.[16]

Slow continuous ultrafiltration (SCUF) may be necessary to augment fluid removal in volume overloaded patients failing to respond to intravenous diuretics.

7.4.2.6 Anticoagulation

Anticoagulation is most frequently achieved using unfractionated heparin as an infusion and monitored hourly using activated clotting times (ACTs). The ACT is a measure of clot formation in whole blood which is not only affected by the degree of anticoagulation, but also clotting factors levels and platelet function and number. A normal ACT is <120–130 s. In most circumstances, the desired ACT while on full ECMO support is 180–200 s. The heparin infusion is stopped transiently or lowered with hemorrhage (ACT 160–180 s) or increased if thrombus is observed in the circuit or lower ECMO flow rates are used (ACT 200–220 s). The monitoring of other coagulation tests and blood count is usually performed at least once or twice daily. In the current era, many centers are routinely using thromboelastography or TEG (see anticoagulation in long-term VAD section). Extreme thrombocytopenia is avoided and platelet transfusion is considered at platelet count of 25–100 k cells/mm^3 depending upon the risk of bleeding and patient population. Fibrinogen is often replaced when ≤75–100 mg/dL.

7.4.3 Complications

The main groups of complications are hemorrhagic, neurologic, and circuit related complications. **Bleeding** is a common complication especially when ECMO is utilized after cardiac surgery. Contributing factors include hemodilution and consumption of clotting factors and platelets, trauma, platelet dysfunction, disseminated intravascular coagulation with fibrinolysis, and anticoagulation. The most common sites of bleeding are surgical sites. When significant hemorrhage occurs, normalization of the platelet count, clotting times, and fibrinogen level is necessary by transfusion of blood products. Aminocaproic acid, an anti-fibrinolytic agent, and more recently recombinant factor VIIa have been used to control bleeding after surgery, but may promote clot formation in the circuit.[21]

Neurologic complications can be devastating and are one of the major reasons for discontinuation of ECMO support. Hemorrhagic or thromboembolic strokes may occur. The highest frequency of neurologic complications is seen in newborns with intracranial hemorrhage occurring in 1 in 10.

Circuit complications can include both mechanical and infectious complications. Mechanical complications related to the circuit occur frequently and include circuit clots, disseminated intravascular coagulation (DIC) related to the circuit, problems with cannula position, or membrane oxygenator failure. Membrane oxygenator failure is often signaled by an increasing pressure gradient across the membrane oxygenator, but may occur suddenly.

Other complications include sepsis and multiorgan failure. The incidence of complications increases with time, thus limiting the use of ECMO for long-term support.

7.4.4 Outcome with Pediatric Cardiac ECMO

The Extracorporeal Life Support Organization (ELSO) was established in 1982, and has been collecting data on ECMO use to support cardio-respiratory failure in children and adults since 1989. Currently 110 centers including 10 international centers contribute data to the registry. The registry database has information on demographics, diagnosis, treatment, and complications. The registry report was recently analyzed with a focus on neonatal and pediatric cardiac cases.[22] As of July 2008, there were 3,416 neonatal and 4,181 pediatric (1 month to 18 years) cardiac ECMO runs reported to the ELSO registry. Survival for cardiac ECMO has remained unchanged over the past decade at approximately 40%. The most common cardiac diagnosis is CHD; 86% in neonates, 79% in children from 1 month to 1 year, and 50% in children from 1 year to 18 years. Survival to discharge for neonatal cardiac ECMO is 38% (compared to 76% for respiratory ECMO), and survival for pediatric cardiac ECMO is 45%.The best outcome is reported for children with acute fulminant myocarditis with survival of 62–67%. According to the registry data, 60% of patients remain on inotropes while on ECMO. Surgical bleeding is quite common and reported in nearly 30% across all age groups, and renal dysfunction requiring hemofiltration is reported in 18–25% of patients. Oxygenator related issues such as clots in the circuit, oxygenator, bladder, or oxygenator failure are also quite common and reported in 18% of neonates, and 15% of older children.

Several single center studies have attempted to identify risk factors for poor outcome for cardiac ECMO (Table 7.3). Presence of significant acidosis prior to initiation of ECMO has been associated with worse survival. This underscores the importance of "urgent" rather than 'emergent" placement of patients on ECMO. For post-cardiotomy patients, longer duration of CPB has been associated with worse outcome. Diagnosis of single ventricle physiology has not been consistently identified as a risk factor (see section on single ventricle). End organ dysfunction particularly renal dysfunction has been predictive of poor outcome on a consistent basis, and so has longer duration of ECMO support.

In a large single center report of cardiac ECMO, 137 patients were supported with ECMO from 1995 to 2001.[23] This represented 2.6% of total admissions to the cardiac intensive care unit; 65% had undergone cardiac surgery. The median age was 4.7 months (1 day–42 years). A majority of patients were placed on ECMO in the post-operative period; 10% failed to separate from CPB, 23% had LCOS refractory to conventional therapy, and 39% required E-CPR. In this series, 39% survived to discharge and risk factors for non-survival included age less than 1 month, male sex, longer period of pre-ECMO mechanical ventilation, and renal and liver dysfunction while on ECMO.

7.4.5 E-CPRO utcomes

The current guidelines from the American Heart Association for Pediatric Advanced Life Support recommend consideration of ECMO for in-hospital cardiac arrest "if the

Table7. 3 ECMOs urvivala ndr iskf actors

Authors	Survival	Riskf actors
Duncan (*1999*) (01/87–05/96)	27/67 (40%)	pH, HCO3, renal failure
Aharon (*2001*) (05/97–10/00)	25/50(50%)	Renal failure, CPB > 45 m, longer duration of ECMO
Kolovos (*2003*) (07/95–06/01)	37/74(50%)	Single ventricle., need for dialysis
Thourani (*2006*) (07/02–02/04)	16/27(59%)	Post-op ventricular failure

condition leading to the arrest is reversible or amenable to heart transplantation". The data from the ELSO registry was recently analyzed for outcomes for patients less than 18 years using E-CPR.[24] From 1992 to 2005, E-CPR was used in 682 patients; the median age of the patients was 3 months,[1,28] and the median weight was 4.6 kg (3.2, 12). CHD was present in 398 of 499 patients with a cardiac diagnosis. 261 patients or 38% survived to discharge. The use of E-CPR increased over 14 years, however survival did not change. By multivariate analysis, cardiac diagnosis and neonatal respiratory diagnosis, white race, and pH > 7.17 were associated with lower odds of mortality. A complicated ECMO course such as persistent acidosis (pH < 7.2), renal dysfunction, pulmonary hemorrhage and neurologic dysfunction predicted mortality. Duration of CPR was not associated with worse survival. Thus, there is clearly a role for E-CPR in select cardiac patients. In institutions with a well established E-CPR program, a patient's candidacy for E-CPR (inpatients) should be discussed on a regular basis so that these difficult decisions are not made emergently, and the ECMO team can be mobilized as expeditiously as possible.

7.5 CentrifugalP ump VAD

Historically, the centrifugal pump has been the mainstay of short-term pediatric VAD support. This device evolved as the need for a mechanical support device superior to conventional ECMO became necessary, especially for patients with isolated ventricular failure. With this VAD, an extracorporeal centrifugal pump produces a vortex continuous nonpulsatile flow, which creates a negative pressure that enables blood to move (Fig. 7.2). The BP-50 and BP-80 models have volumes of 50 and 80 mL respectively. Heparin-bonded tubing can be used to minimize the need for anticoagulation. Compared to roller pumps, there is less trauma to red blood cells and less pronounced inflammatory response. Cannulation is performed via the left atrium and aorta (left ventricular assist) or right

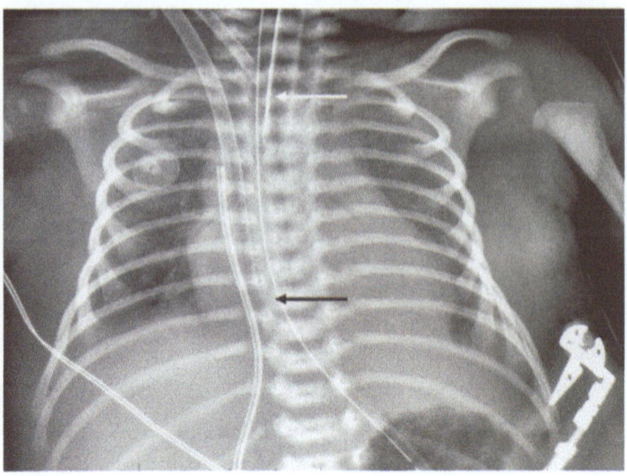

Fig.7. 2 Ac hestra diograph of a patient on VA ECMO. The white arrow demonstrates the arterial cannula tip and the black arrow the venousc annulat ip

atrium and pulmonary artery (right ventricular assist). Advantages include its ease of implantation, fast set-up time, and low priming volume, low-level anticoagulation, and lower cost. Disadvantages include its shorter duration of usage, occasional thrombus in the circuit as well as its nonpulsatile flow.

Thuys and associates reported the use of the Biopump (Medtronic Bio-Medicus, Minneapolis, MN) in 34 children with an average age of 60 days (2–258 days), and average weight of 3.7 kg (1.9–5.98 kg). Sixty-three percent of patients were successfully decannulated from VAD support and 31% survived to hospital discharge.[25] The Royal Children's Hospital in Australia has had an extensive experience with a centrifugal pump VAD.[26] From 1989–2005, 116 infants and children underwent centrifugal pump VAD support. This cohort constituted about 1% of the CPB cases performed during that time. Median age was 3.0 months (2 days to 19 years) and the median weight was 4.6 kg (1.9–70). The probability of weaning the patients from VAD was 66% (confidence limits 56–75%). The probability of hospital discharge was 43% (confidence limits 31–55%). The median support time was 75 h (range 19–428 h).

7.6 Long-term Ventricular Assist Devices

The pediatric experience with long-term VAD has been growing especially since the availability of pulsatile devices in miniaturized versions. Advantages of these devices include their chronic support capability, ease of use, capability for biventricular support without an oxygenator, mobility for cardiac rehabilitation, need for low-level anticoagulation, and pulsatile flow nature with the pulsatile devices. Disadvantages include a propensity to have thromboembolic complications, difficulty of implantation/explantation, cumulative cost, exteriorization of the cannulae (paracorporeal devices), increased risk of pre-sensitization (elevated panel reactive antibody titers), and size limitation especially with biventricular support. Infection is also a serious complication, the risk of which can be minimized by immobilization of the driveline as close to the exit site as possible with a binder.

7.6.1 Contraindications and Special Considerations

Placement of long-term VAD is contraindicated in patients with severe neurologic injury, uncontrolled coagulopathy, and sepsis. Significant aortic regurgitation will interfere with forward flow from a left ventricular assist device; this problem can be overcome by closing the leaflets as long as the tissue is robust. A pre-existing mechanical prosthetic valve may become frozen shut with thrombus, thus becoming a risk for thromboembolic complication. A VAD seems to function normally in the absence of a mitral valve, so one can consider removing a prosthetic mitral valve.

Table 7.1 lists the available long-term devices in the USA.

The Berlin heart is a paracorporeal pneumatically driven pulsatile device that has been available for use in a miniaturized version since 1992. The inlet is cannulation via the ventricular apex or atrium, and the outlet is to the aorta or pulmonary artery with both cannulas exteriorized. The polyurethane pumps have a wide range of stroke volumes of 10, 25, 30, 50, 60, or 80 mL (Figs. 7.3 and 7.4). Three membranes provide stability and the system is heparin coated. Silicon cannulas connect the blood pump to the patient. The pumps are driven by a pulsatile pneumatic system. The blood pumps have a transparent polyurethane housing which divides an air chamber and blood chamber by a triple layer

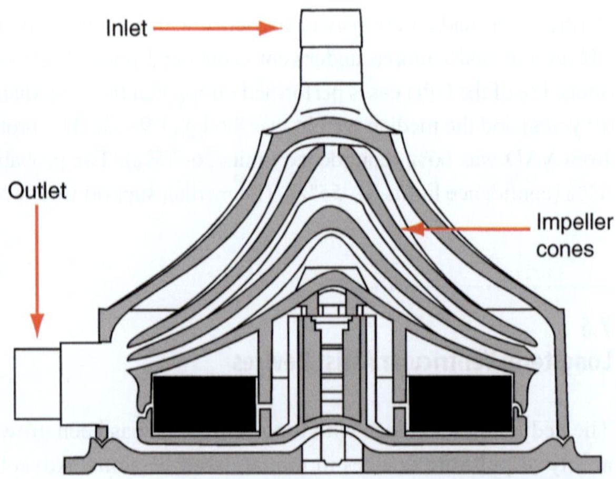

Fig. 7.3 Berlin Heart Pump (inlet, outlet and impeller cones)

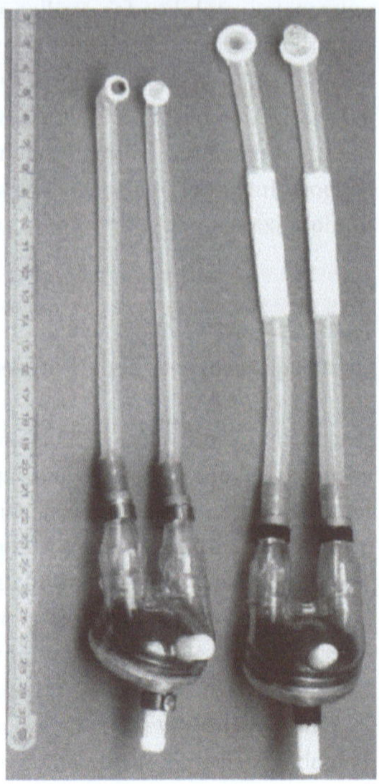

Fig. 7.4 Two different sizes of Berlin Heart pumps

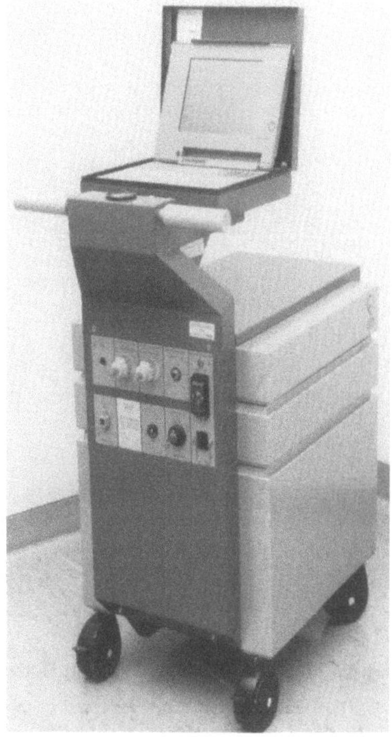

Fig. 7.5 BerlinH eartC onsole

membrane. In pump diastole, blood is drawn into the blood chamber by negative pressure in the air chamber, and in pump systole, the air chamber is inflated thus pushing blood out of the blood chamber (Fig. 7.6). A rechargeable battery can provide up to 5 h of independent power supply. This device can provide univentricular support (right or left) or biventricular support. Early complication of thrombus formation has been lessened with the use of heparin-coated system (Carmeda Inc., Texas). This device has been successfully used in infants as a bridge to transplantation (Fig. 7.7).

The ***MEDOS HIA*** VAD is another pulsatile, paracorporeal pneumatically driven VAD with limited pediatric experience in Europe.

The paracorporeal nature of these devices allows for extubation and ambulation. The clear polyurethane pump housing allows thrombus to be readily visualized, leading to pump change if it persists despite more aggressive anti-coagulation. There is an ongoing prospective multicenter Investigational Device Exemption (IDE) study in North America to study the safety and efficacy of the Berlin heart EXCOR device. The device is approved by the FDA for compassionate use to non-IDE sites. This device has been used in >200 children in North America.

The ***Thoratec*** is a pneumatically powered pulsatile VAD that consists of a flexible seam-free segmented sac within a ridged polycarbonate housing (Fig. 7.8). There are tilting disc valves in the inlet and outlet portions. The inlet is cannulation via the left atrium or ventricular apex and the outlet is to the aorta with both cannulas exteriorized. Cannulation of the left ventricular apex is preferred due to reduced risk of thromboembolism. An

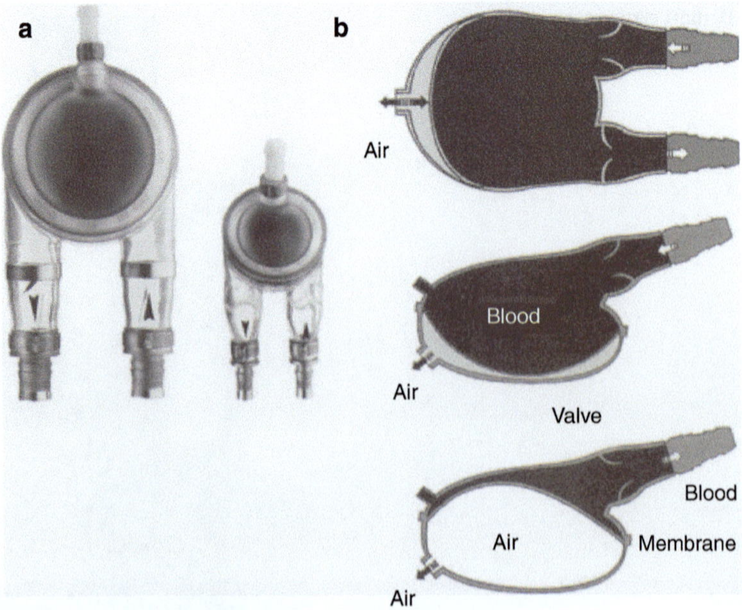

Fig. 7.6 Berlinhe art(M odified from Hetzer et al.[30]W ithpe rmission)

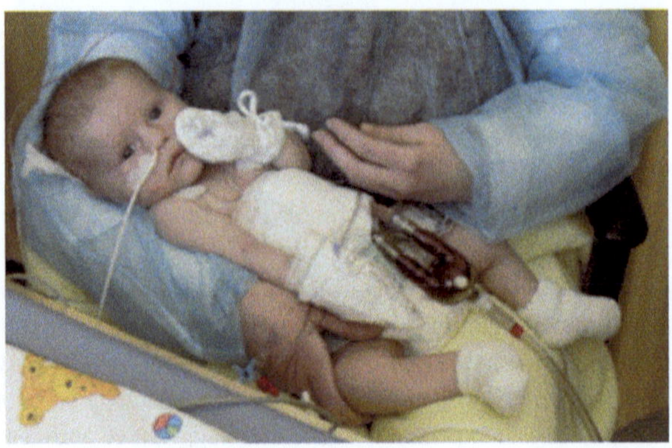

Fig. 7.7 Infant with Berlin Heart Devicei npl ace

exception is patients with restrictive cardiomyopathy in whom atrial cannulation may be preferred as the ventricles are usually hypertrophied but not dilated. The stroke volume is 65 mL with a maximum output of 7 L/min. This device is suitable for older children (>30 kg). Three modes exist: fixed rate, synchronous, or volume. Once patients are extubated and stable, the large console can be replaced by a portable one which is the size of a small suitcase. This allows for ambulation and rehabilitation (Fig. 7.9).

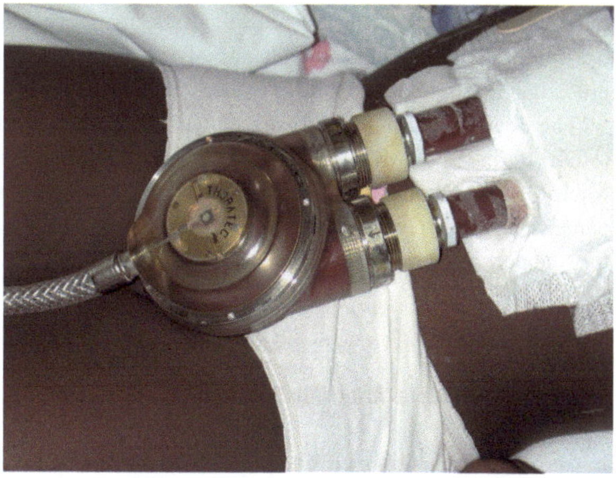

Fig. 7.8 Thoratec device in place

7.6.2
Axial-Flow Devices

Although the pediatric experience with axial-flow devices such as the DeBakey device is limited to a few adolescents, its smaller size holds promise for future pediatric use.[27] This class of devices consists of relatively small axial pumps that involve an impeller with its housing that is entirely implantable. The advantages of such an axial system are the relative ease of implantation, decreased infection, and its continuous flow provides unloading throughout the cardiac cycle. Its disadvantages are the need for a large-sized ventricular apical cannulation, and higher incidence of hemolysis.

The **MicroMed DeBakey** is a small titanium axial device with inflow from the left ventricle and outflow to the ascending aorta pushing blood at 7,500–12,500 rpm and up to 10 L/min (see Fig. 7.10). This was the first long-term axial flow circulatory assist device

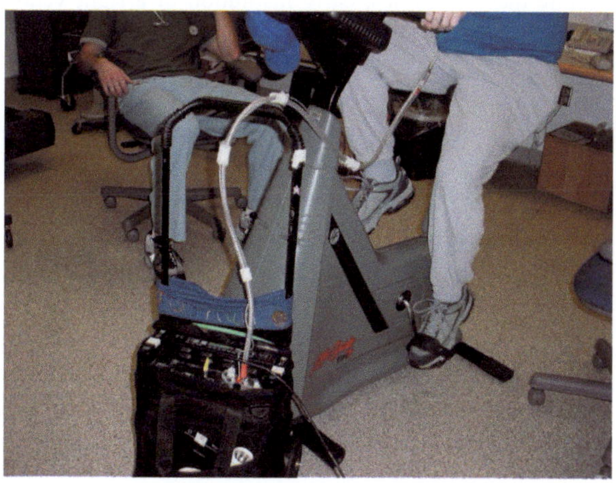

Fig. 7.9 Portable Thoratec device

to be introduced as a bridge to transplant. Its small size makes it potentially attractive for use in children. Potential advantages of this device include ease of implantation, and unloading throughout the cardiac cycle.

The Food and Drug Administration (FDA) granted a humanitarian device exemption (HDE) to the MicroMed DeBakey VAD Child in 2004. As a condition of that approval, MicroMed was mandated to collect data in a systematic fashion for the first 50 pediatric patients, aged 5–16 years old, with BSA ≥ 0.7 and < 1.5 m^2 who need mechanical circulatory support as a bridge to cardiac transplantation.

7.6.3 Management Principles After VAD Placement

In the immediate post-operative period after VAD implantation, patients on VAD need to be fully ventilated and oxygenated. It is also important to remember that output from the VAD is dependent on preload and afterload. Although most children with end-stage cardiomyopathy or congenital heart disease have biventricular dysfunction, the ventricular unloading provided by the "left" or "systemic" VAD has generally made the need for biventricular assist uncommon. It is important to appreciate that the right ventricular output is the preload to the left ventricular assist device (LVAD). Inadequate filling of the LVAD may be from low intravascular volume, tamponade, right ventricular dysfunction, pulmonary hypertension, or arrhythmias. Monitoring of central venous pressure is critical in these patients, and there should be frequent echocardiographic assessment of right ventricular function and right ventricular pressure. Right ventricular dysfunction and elevated pulmonary vascular resistance need to be treated in a timely fashion with inspired nitric oxide or pharmacological agents such as milrinone, isoproterenol, or occasionally prostacycline. Inotropic support with dopamine and/or epinephrine may be required to support the right ventricle especially in the early postoperative period after LVAD placement. Patients who remain dependent on inspired nitric oxide can be transitioned to oral sildenafil as a pulmonary vasodilator. If pulmonary hypertension persists despite these therapies, early institution of a right ventricular assist device should be considered.

7.6.3.1 Anticoagulation for VAD

Heparin is used in the immediate post-operative period once bleeding is well controlled. The goal activated PTT time is 60–85 s. Addition of Aspirin should be deferred until the platelet count has stabilized, and bleeding is well under control. Long-term anticoagulation can be maintained with warfarin (goal INR 2.5–3.5) or low molecular weight heparin (target antifactor Xa level 0.5–1) in combination with anti-platelet agents such as aspirin, dipyridamole or clopidogrel. A more aggressive approach may be indicated in cases where thrombus accumulates in the pump head. This may even necessitate replacement of the pump with the Berlin heart device. The widespread utilization of VADs in children has highlighted the pitfalls associated with traditional monitoring of anticoagulation with activated PTT. Additional monitoring is now frequently utilized and includes measurement of antifactor Xa levels (target is 0.35–0.5 for unfractionated heparin), antithrombin III levels and use of thromboelastography or TEG. If adequate anticoagulation is not achieved despite up titration of heparin, fresh frozen plasma is recommended to maintain antithrombin III level >70%. Platelet aggregation tests are also performed to monitor antiplatelet activity.

7.6.4 Complications

Like ECMO, complications include bleeding, neurological complications, thromboembolic complications, sepsis, and multiorgan failure (discussed in outcomes). Other adverse events include pancreatitis, and arrhythmias. Arrhythmias are quite common after VAD placement. Persistent arrhythmia warrants treatment with a LVAD, since right ventricular output which is the preload to the LVAD may be compromised.

7.6.5 Outcome with Pediatric VAD

7.6.5.1 MEDOS HIA

Survival with this device has been reported to be 36.2% in children up to 16 years of age, including an infant with a body surface area less than 0.3 m^2. Konertz and associates described a series of 6 children supported with this device.[28] The patients' age ranged from 5 days to 8 years, and their weight ranged from 3.1 to 20 kg. Aspirin and heparin were used for anticoagulation. Four of six patients (67%) survived to discharge, two patients were bridged to transplantation, and two were weaned from the device.

7.6.5.2 Berlin Heart

These devices have been available in a miniaturized version in Europe since the 1990s. Ishino and associates reported the use of the Berlin heart in 14 children with an average age of 1 month (2 weeks to 15 years) and average weight of 14.9 kg (3.2–52 kg). Complications included mediastinal exploration for bleeding in six patients, and three pump changes for thrombus visualized in the pump.[29] Eight patients were transplanted with four survivors, and three were decannulated due to recovery of ventricular function with one survivor.

Hetzer and colleagues reported their experience with the use of the Berlin heart EXCOR device in 62 children from 1990 to 2004.[30] This study included 10 children with end stage heart failure from CHD, and 14 children with CHD who required VAD support after CPB. Survival for the whole group improved from 35% in the 1990s to 68% from 2000–2004. This was mostly due to better survival in children with a diagnosis of cardiomyopathy (43% versus 76%) and post-cardiotomy support (none versus 57%). Survival improved in infants as well with 78% survival from 2000–2004 as opposed to no survival in the previous decade (Figs. 7.11 and 7.12). Modifications made from the 1990s to the more recent years include less frequent use of biventricular assist, earlier institution of VAD support before development of irreversible end organ dysfunction or circulatory collapse, heparin coating of blood pumps, alteration in cannulae, and addition of anti-platelet therapy such as aspirin/dipyridamole and more aggressive monitoring of anticoagulation.

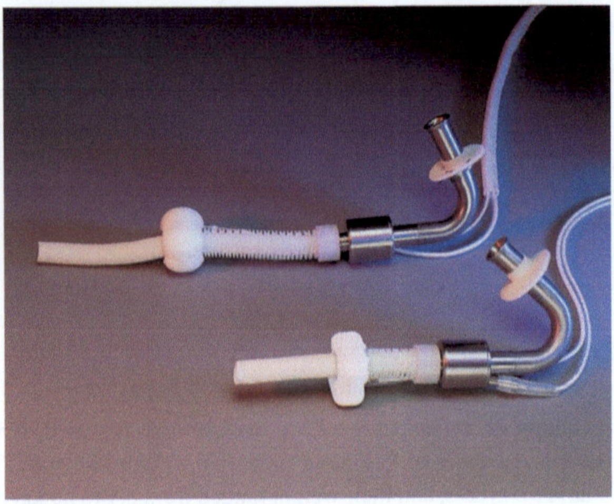

Fig.7.10 MicroMed DeBakeya xialde vice

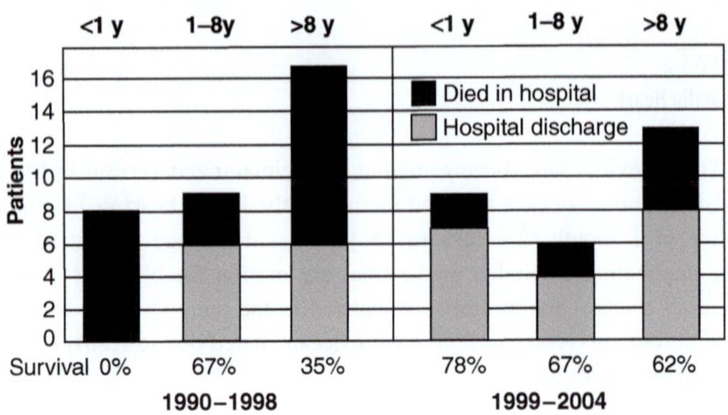

Fig.7.11 Survivalby age (Modified from Hetzer et al.[30] Withpe rmission)

7.6.5.3 The Thoratec VAD

In a large series of 209 pediatric patients supported with the Thoratec device, survival was 68%.[31] Mean age was 14.5 years (5–18 years), mean weight was 57 kg (17–118 kg), and mean body surface area was 1.6 m^2 (0.7–2.3 m^2). Indications for mechanical circulatory support included cardiomyopathy in 55%, myocarditis in 25%, and end-stage congenital heart disease in 6% of patients. The average duration of support was 44 days (0–434 days). Survival rates were higher for patients with myocarditis (86%), cardiomyopathy (74%), compared with patients with congenital heart disease (27%). On performing a sub analysis of children with body surface area of less than 1.3 m^2, there was a higher proportion of children with congenital heart disease.[32] The smallest child in this series was 17 kg with a body surface area of 0.7 m^2. Survival for this group was 52%. Neurological complications were significant in the congenital heart disease group and also more commonly associated with cannulation of the left atrium.

The Pediatric Heart Transplant Study (PHTS) group data was recently analyzed to evaluate the outcome of pediatric patients <18 years of age who were bridged to heart transplantation with VAD support.[33] Of 2,375 patients listed for heart transplantation from 1993 to 2003, VAD was implanted in 99 children. Median age was 13.3 years (2 days to 17.9 years) and median weight was 56 kg (3–150 kg). 21/99 had a diagnosis of CHD; five children had a diagnosis of single ventricle, five had L-Transposition of great arteries (TGA), three had critical aortic stenosis, and eight patients required VAD support after cardiotomy. The Thoratec was the most frequently used device in 53 patients. It is worth noting that only one patient was supported with the Berlin heart during the study period. The median duration of support was 25 days ([1]–465). Seventy-seven children were successfully bridged to transplantation, and five recovered myocardial function and were decannulated. Risk factors for death prior to transplant included a diagnosis of CHD, female sex, and earlier era. Common complications included bleeding and infection in a third of patients each, and neurologic complications in nearly a fifth of patients. Hemolysis occurred in 19 patients, and multiorgan failure in 2 patients. In this large multiinstitutional study, VAD support prior to transplantation did not affect 5-year survival after transplantation (Fig. 7.13).

In another single center study, 20 patients were supported with pulsatile VAD of the systemic ventricle (LVAD in 18) from 1998 to 2008.[34] The median age was 14.3 years (3 months to 25 years). The Thoratec was the most frequently used device in 14 patients. Four patients had refractory ventricular dysfunction due to CHD remote from surgery; one with L-TGA late after the Rastelli operation, one with congenital mitral stenosis after placement of mitral and aortic prosthetic valves, one with tricuspid atresia with a failing Fontan, and one with D-TGA late after the Mustard operation. Thus in 2/4 patients with CHD, the systemic right ventricle was supported with a VAD. Median duration of support was 67 days (11–424). 17/20 patients were extubated. Fourteen patients were successfully bridged to transplant, and one recovered myocardial function. Of the five deaths, two occurred in patients with CHD.

The **Heartmate** V-E is a pulsatile implantable VAD that has been used in older children. Helman et al. described the use of this device in 12 adolescents (body surface area of

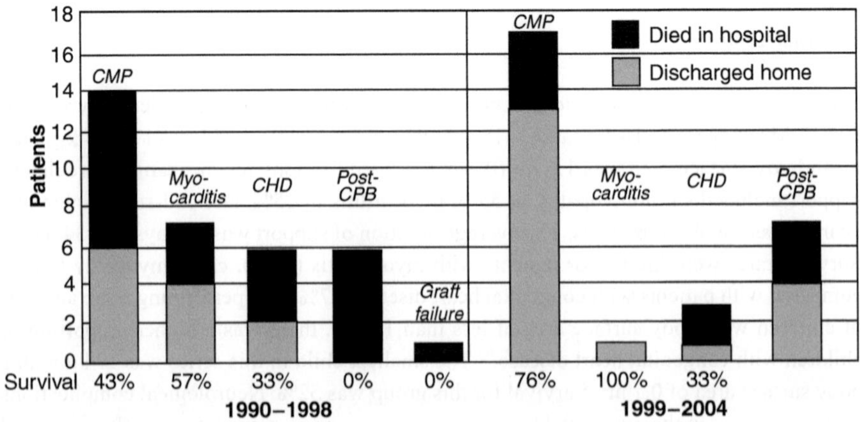

Fig.7.12 Survival by diagnosis (Modified from Hetzer et al.[30] W ithpe rmission)

1.4–2.2 m^2); a majority of these patients had a dilated cardiomyopathy. As in the adult population, the majority of children supported with the vented electrical model was discharged home and resumed normal activity.[35]

The **DeBakey child** axial device was FDA approved for HDE use in children in 2004. However the use of this device has been limited due to complications such as bleeding from erosion at the site of implantation of the device. The availability of the Berlin heart VAD may have also contributed to limited utilization of the DeBakey child. The Berlin heart EXCOR device IDE study was started more or less at the same time, and the device has been available for compassionate use as well.

7.6.6 VAD and Pre-sensitization

Several studies have reported a higher incidence of pre-sensitization or development of antibodies against human leukocyte antigen (HLA) among adults supported with VAD. Proposed risk factors for pre-sensitization include exposure to multiple blood products, prior surgeries, and the immune activating property of the specific VAD and the circuit. The incidence of VAD associated pre-sensitization was recently described in a single center pediatric study.[34] Nineteen of the twenty patients had a negative panel reactive antibody (PRA) before VAD implantation. PRA data was not available in three patients who died before transplantation. Six patients became pre-sensitized before transplantation, representing 35% of the patients. Five of six patients remained pre-sensitized after transplantation; however this was transient in two patients. The remaining three patients continue to have high anti-HLA antibodies at a mean follow-up of 2.29 ± 1.1 years, with two patients having donor-specific antibodies. Pre-sensitization on VAD did not affect the incidence of rejection or survival. In this study, black race was the only risk factor associated with pre-sensitization. As the use of VAD support continues to expand in children, it is important to serially measure PRA both before and after transplantation.

7.6.7 Mechanical Circulatory Support in Patients with Single Ventricle Physiology

A majority of children with single ventricle physiology undergo a three-staged reconstruction to achieve completion of the Fontan circulation. The syndrome of low cardiac output is quite common in this population through all three stages of reconstruction, and some of these patients will eventually require cardiac transplantation. While conventional therapy with inotropic support and afterload reduction remains the mainstay of therapy for the failing heart in these children, there is a role for mechanical support in select patients. Most of this experience is limited to the use of ECMO.

7.6.7.1 Special Considerations in "Shunt Dependent" Patients on ECMO

It is possible to use a standardized circuit, including a servo-regulated system driven by a roller pump or a centrifugal pump, for mechanical support in the "shunt dependent" patient. In the late 1980s and early 1990s, it was a common practice to ligate the shunt while on ECMO. In a study performed in 20 piglets on CPB, the main pulmonary artery was ligated in 10 thus eliminating pulmonary blood flow, and antegrade pulmonary blood flow was maintained in the remaining piglets on CPB.[36] At the end of the experiment, all 20 piglets had significant lung disease with increased alveolar-arterial gradient, poor lung compliance and increase in pulmonary vascular resistance. These findings were exaggerated in the piglets in whom the main pulmonary artery was ligated on CPB. Based on this experiment, clinical practice was changed. In a study of ECMO in 35 postcardiotomy patients over a 5-year period, nine patients were "shunt dependent".[36] The shunt was ligated in the first four patients in this study, and there were no survivors. Autopsies performed in 2/4 patients revealed pulmonary infarcts. The shunt was left open in the subsequent five patients, and 4/5 survived. It is now common practice to leave the aorto-pulmonary shunt open while on ECMO. ECMO flows and sweep gas are adjusted to maintain adequate systemic blood pressure, tissue perfusion, and gas exchange. Due to significant runoff through the shunt towards the pulmonary circulation, some patients may require flows as high as 150–200 mL/kg/min. In a majority of patients, the membrane can be isolated, and the circuit utilized as a ventricular assist device or "no membrane oxygenator" or NOMO ECMO (Fig. 7.14). Potential advantages include less inflammation, and requirement of lower level of anticoagulation.

Fig. 7. 13 (Modified from Blume et al.[33] W ith permission)

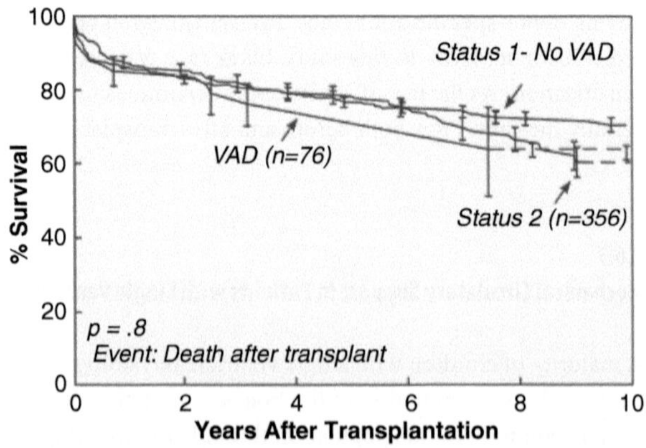

7.6.7.2
Outcome of ECMO in "Shunt Dependent" Single Ventricle Patients

The registry of the Extracorporeal Life Support Organization reported the outcome of extracorporeal support for neonates with cardiac indications from 1996 to 2000.[37] The registry recorded 740 neonates who were placed on extracorporeal life support for cardiac indications at less than 30 days. There were 118 neonates with hypoplastic left heart syndrome (HLHS). There was no significant difference in survival between patients with HLHS compared with other defects. For those with HLHS, placement on extracorporeal life support at greater than 15 days of age was significantly associated with better survival. For the whole group, placement on extracorporeal life support at less than 3 days of age was significantly associated with better survival. Survivors also had a shorter duration of support.

A recent report reviewed a large single center's experience with "non-elective" extracorporeal membrane oxygenation after the Norwood operation for HLHS and its variants over a period of 7.5 years.[38] Of the 382 infants who underwent the Norwood operation during the study period, 34 or 9.4% required ECMO in the post-operative period. Indications for ECMO included inability to separate from CPB in 14 infants, and cardiopulmonary arrest due to circulatory failure or severe hypoxemia in 22. Of this group, almost two-fifths (38.8%) survived to hospital discharge or transfer. Longer duration of CPB, the need for ECMO early in the post-operative period, and longer duration of support were associated with worse survival. All five infants who had a cardiac arrest due to shunt thrombosis survived, as opposed to one-third of those arresting due to other causes. The mean duration of support was significantly less for those who survived. As with the report from the registry, there was a trend toward a longer time to ECMO after the Norwood operation among survivors. Of the early survivors, half of the infants are alive at a median follow-up of 20 months. In another study of ECMO in 44 "shunt dependent" patients, survival to hospital discharge was 50%.[39] Similar to the previous study, the probability of survival was better in patients with "hypoxemia" as an indication for ECMO rather than "circulatory collapse". Thus predictors of poor outcome after ECMO in "shunt dependent" single ventricle patients include circulatory collapse rather than hypoxemia/shunt thrombosis as the indication for ECMO, and requirement of ECMO in the immediate post-operative period after the Norwood operation.

Ungerleider and co-workers have suggested that mechanical support should be routine after the Norwood operation, arguing that this approach simplifies post-operative management and improves hospital survival.[40] They have used their protocol in 18 consecutive patients undergoing the Norwood operation, with a mean duration of mechanical support of 3 ± 0.1 days. Survival to discharge was 87%, with improved early neurodevelopmental outcomes. Such routine mechanical support after the Norwood operation is a novel approach that addresses the increased cardiac output demands in the immediate post-operative period, and as argued, simplifies post-operative care. The approach, nonetheless, will likely increase cost and the need for additional support personnel.

7.6.7.3 ECMO in Cavopulmonary Connections

There is very limited experience with mechanical support in patients with cavopulmonary connections. The registry of Extracorporeal Life Support reported survival in 25% of patients with this physiology. The largest experience reported is a series of 20 patients with cavopulmonary connections supported with ECMO from 1984 to 2002.[41] In patients with a bidirectional Glenn, only one of six patients survived, and this patient sustained severe neurological damage. In those with the Fontan circulation, half survived to discharge, and one-third are alive at follow-up. This report highlights some of the technical difficulties in this challenging group of patients. Patients with cavopulmonary connections are difficult to resuscitate effectively with conventional cardiopulmonary resuscitation. During resuscitation, the increase in intrathoracic pressure may restrict effective flow of blood to the lungs and oxygenation, as well as increasing cerebral venous pressure that may further limit cerebral perfusion. This obviously increases the risk of neurologic injury. This study also demonstrates the inability to maintain adequate venous drainage and systemic perfusion in these patients, and the frequent need for multiple venous cannulae in patients with Fontanc irculation.

7.6.7.4 VAD and Single Ventricle Patients

There are isolated case reports of use of VAD in patients with single ventricle physiology. In "shunt dependent" single ventricle patients, the ECMO circuit can be used as a VAD without a membrane oxygenator (see previous section). However this is usually not a viable long term option for these infants as a bridge to transplantation. There is a growing population of children and young adults with "Fontan failure". The causes of heart failure in this patient population include ventricular dysfunction (systolic and diastolic), arrhythmias, and protein losing enteropathy. Many of these patients have a chronic low output state with elevated venous pressure. In addition these patients frequently have unrecognized renal and liver dysfunction, and in general are high risk transplant candidates. They obviously lack a

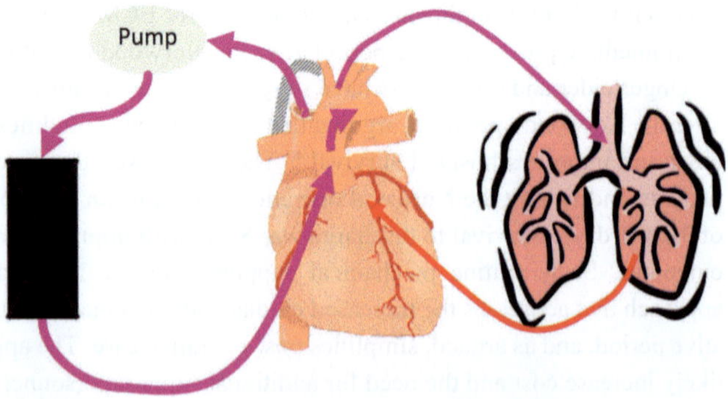

Fig. 7. 14 Isolation of membrane oxygenator in parallel pulmonary circulation

"sub-pulmonary ventricle", and their anatomy and physiology pose unique challenges with regard to VAD placement. Surgeons have been quite innovative in an attempt to support a handful of these patients with a VAD.[42] For example, one approach includes disconnecting the inferior vena cava (IVC) from the extracardiac conduit and the superior vena cava (SVC) from the pulmonary artery, using a new chamber between the SVC and IVC for inflow cannulation of the VAD, and using the extracardiac conduit for outflow cannulation (Fig. 7.15). Notwithstanding these innovations, there are no long term survivors.

In an attempt to add a sub-pulmonary ventricle, investigators have proposed use of a "pump" such as an impeller or axial device within the Fontan circuit.[43–45] However, these studies are in a pre-clinical stage and not ready for testing in humans yet.

7.6.8 Long-term Follow-up of Survivors of Mechanical Circulatory Support

In a recent report, 37 children (26 ECMO and 11 VAD survivors) were followed for an average of more than 4 years.[46] Only one patient died in either group for an overall long-term survival of 95%. Eighty percent of children in both groups were reportedly in excellent general condition, and ventricular function by echocardiographic evaluation was normal in all the ECMO survivors and in 90% of the VAD survivors. More than 60% of ECMO supported children had moderate to severe neurologic impairment, whereas only 20% of the VAD survivors demonstrated the same degree of neurologic impairment. These results may suggest an advantage for VAD support possibly because of decreased requirements for anticoagulation with less risk for intracranial hemorrhage. However these results must be interpreted with caution as the ECMO-supported group had a higher proportion of critically ill neonates with more complex underlying cardiac conditions.

The largest single center experience with the Berlin heart EXCOR device in North America was recently reported.[47] Over a 4-year period, 17 VADs were impanted in 17 children with refractory ventricular dysfunction as a bridge to transplantation; LVAD in 14 and a biventricular assist device in 3 patients. Three patients had a diagnosis of CHD. Neurologic complications occurred in 7/17 or nearly 40% of patients 8 ± 7 days after VAD implantation. Two of these patients had severe intracranial hemorrhage, and five had thromboembolic events. Two patients died, and among the five survivors, minimal neurologic deficits were noted on short-term follow-up. It is also worth noting that thrombus was not noted in the device or cannula in any of these patients, and there were no changes noted in hematologic parameters at the time of the stroke. The PHTS study reported neurologic events in nearly 20% of patients. Similar to other children with CHD, the long-term neurodevelopmental outcomes of VAD survivors will need to be followed as well.

7.7 A Comparison of ECMO Versus VAD Support

Despite recent advances in VAD technology, ECMO remains the most common mechanical circulatory system in use for pediatric patients. The advantages of ECMO include its familiarity among practitioners, ability to provide biventricular support and respiratory support, universal availability across all pediatric age groups, and relative low cost. Unlike adults in whom pure left ventricular failure is the common indication for mechanical support, cardiopulmonary support is more commonly required in children due to a combination of pulmonary dysfunction, pulmonary hypertension, and right ventricular dysfunction, particularly in the immediate post-operative period. ECMO is obviously the mechanical circulatory support of choice for rapid deployment during cardiopulmonary arrest. (Table 7.4). There are a number of disadvantages, including the need for a dedicated team of ECMO specialists, immobilization, and requirement for intensive care monitoring, risks of bleeding, thrombosis, infection, and multiorgan failure. These attendant disadvantages increase over time and limit the use of ECMO for long-term support.

The advantages of long-term VAD include less trauma to blood cells (lack of membrane oxygenator), and decreased risk of infection compared to ECMO where the system is more open with multiple access ports. Implantable VADs allow greater mobility for cardiac rehabilitation and have chronic support capability as bridge to transplantation. The disadvantages of VAD include the need for transthoracic cannulation, while ECMO can be initiated with peripheral cannulation. In addition biventricular support with VAD requires four cannulas, whereas ECMO provides biventricular support with two cannulas.

Table 7.4 ECMO versus VAD

	ECMO	VAD
Pediatric experience	√	
Simplicity of circuit		√
Peripheral cannulation	√	
LV decompression		√
Biventricular support	√	
Hypoxemia, Pulmonary hypertension	√	
E-CPR	√	

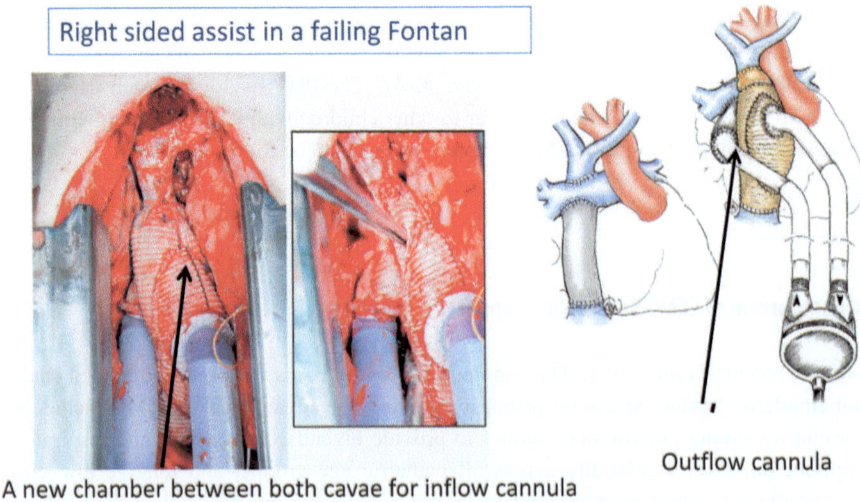

Fig. 7.15 Example of ventricular assist device in failing Fontan circulation

7.8 Future Directions and Conclusion

Experience with mechanical circulatory assist devices in infants and children is increasing with improvement in clinical results. With the introduction of miniaturized assist devices, it is now possible to provide VAD support across all pediatric age groups. VAD support should be instituted "urgently" rather than emergently before the onset of circulatory collapse or irreversible end organ dysfunction. Currently, there is an NHLBI sponsored development effort to design and perform clinical testing of new pediatric devices with most of the proposed systems utilizing the axial flow design. Five devices are currently in preclinical stage of development. INTERMACS or the Interagency Registry for Mechanically Assisted Circulatory Support is a national registry for adults and children receiving a mechanical circulatory support device that was established in 2006. This is a joint effort between the NHLBI, the Center for Medicare and Medicaid Services, the FDA, clinicians, scientists and industry representatives. Data analysis is expected to facilitate better patient evaluation and management, while aiding in better device development. As the overall survival of children with CHD improves, the indications for device placement are likely to increase in the long-term. This includes a growing population of patients with single ventricle physiology developing "heart failure" through all stages of Fontan completion. These patients are anatomically challenging. Many of these patients are "high-risk" candidates for heart transplantation both medically and psychosocially, and one may speculate that VAD support will be available for this patient population in the not so distant future and perhaps "destination therapy" will be an option as well.

References

1. Kanter KR, Pennington DG, Weber TR et al. Extracorporeal membrane oxygenation for postoperative cardiac support in children. *J Thorac Cardiovasc Surg.*1987; 93:27–35.
2. Nido PJ. Extracorporeal membrane oxygenation for cardiac support in children. *Ann Thorac Surg.*1996;61:336–339.
3. Kulik TJ, Moler FW, Palmisano JM et al. Outcome-associated factors in pediatric patients treated with extracorporeal membrane oxygenator after cardiac surgery. *Circulation.* 1996;94: II63–II68.
4. Aharon AS, Drinkwater DC, Churchwell KB et al. Extracorporeal membrane oxygenation in children after repair of congenital cardiac lesions. *Ann Thorac Surg.*2001; 72:2095–2101.
5. Kolovos NS, Bratton SL, Moler FW et al. Outcome of pediatric patients treated with extracorporeal life support after cardiac surgery. *Ann Thorac Surg.* 2003;76:1435–1441; discussion 1441–1442.
6. Bartlett RJ, Gazzaniga AB, Jefferies MR et al. Extracorporeal membrane oxygenation (ECMO) cardiopulmonary support in infancy. *Trans Am Soc Artif Intern Organs.* 1976;22: 80–93.
7. Dalton HJ, Rycus PT, Conrad SA. Update on extracorporeal life support 2004. *Semin Perinatol.* February2005;29(1) :24–33.
8. Duncan BW, Hraska V, Jonas RA et al. Mechanical circulatory support in children with cardiac disease. *J Thorac Cardiovasc Surg.*1999; 117:529–542.
9. Duncan BW. Mechanical circulatory support for infants and children with cardiac disease. *Ann Thorac Surg.*2002; 73:1670–1677.
10. Chang AC, McKenzie ED. Mechanical cardiopulmonary support in children and young adults: Extracorporeal membrane oxygenation, ventricular assist devices, and long-term support devices. *Pediatr Cardiol.*2005; 26:2–28.
11. Luciani GB, Chang AC, Starnes VA. Surgical repair of transposition of great arteries in neonates with persistent pulmonary hypertension. *Ann Thorac Surg.*1996; 61:800–805.
12. Walker GM, McLeod K, Brown KL et al. Extracorporeal life support as a treatment of supraventricular tachycardia in infants. *Pediatr Crit Care Med.*2003; 4:52–54.
13. Cohen MI, Gaynor JW, Ramesh V et al. Extracorporeal membrane oxygenation for patients with refractory ventricular arrhythmias. *J Thorac Cardiovasc Surg.*1999; 118:961–963.
14. di Russo GB, Clark BJ, Bridges ND et al. Prolonged extracorporeal membrane oxygenation as a bridge to cardiac transplantation. *Ann Thorac Surg.*2000; 69:925–927.
15. del Nido PJ, Duncan BW, Meyer JE et al. Left ventricular assist device improves survival in children with left ventricular dysfunction after repair of anomalous origin of the left coronary artery from the pulmonary artery. *Ann Thorac Surg.*1999; 67:169–172.
16. Del Nido PJ, Dalton HJ, Thomson AE, Siewers RD. Extracorporeal membrane oxygenator rescue in children during cardiac arrest after cardiac surgery. *Circulation.* 1992;86: II300–II304.
17. Duncan BW, Ibrahim AE, Hraska V et al. Use of rapid-deployment extracorporeal membrane oxygenation for the resuscitation of pediatric patients with heart disease after cardiac arrest. *J Thorac Cardiovasc Surg.*1998; 116:305–311.
18. Jacobs JP, Ojito JW, McConaghey TW et al. Rapid cardiopulmonary support for children with complex congenital heart disease. *Ann Thorac Surg.*200 0;70:742–750.
19. Hetzer R, Loebe M, Potapov EV et al. Circulatory support with pneumatic paracorporeal ventricular assist device in infants and children. *Ann Thorac Surg.*1998; 66:1498–1506.
20. Koenig PR, Ralston MA, Kimball TR et al. Balloon atrial septostomy for left ventricular decompression in patients receiving extracorporeal membrane oxygenation for myocardial failure. *J Pediatr.*1993; 122:S95–S99.

21. Dominguez TE, Mitchell M, Friess SH et al. Use of recombinant factor VIIa for refractory hemorrhage during extracorporeal membrane oxygenation. *Pediatr Crit Care Med.* 2005; 6:348–351.
22. Haines NM, Rycus PT, Zwischenberger JB et al. Extracorporeal Life Support Registry Report 2008: neonatal and pediatric cardiac cases. *ASAIO J.*2 009;55:111–116.
23. Morris MC, Ittenbach RF, Godinez RI et al. Risk factors for mortality in 137 pediatric cardiac intensive care unit patients managed with extracorporeal membrane oxygenation. *Crit Care Med.*2004;32:1061–1069.
24. Thiagarajan RR, Laussen PC, Rycus PT et al. Extracorporeal membrane oxygenation to aid cardiopulmonary resuscitation in infants and children. *Circulation.*2007; 116:1693–1700.
25. Thuys CA, Mullaly RJ, Horton SB et al. Centrifugal ventricular assist in children under 6 kg. *Euro J Cardiothorac Surg.*1998; 13:130–134.
26. Karl TR, Horton SB. Centrifugal pump VAD in pediatric cardiac surgery. In: Duncan BW, ed. *Mechanical Circulatory Support for Pediatric Cardiac Patients.* New York, NY: Marcel Dekker;2001:21 –48.
27. Wieselthaler GM, Schima H, Hiesmayr M et al. First clinical experience with the DeBakey VAD continuous-axial-flow pump for bridge to transplantation. *Circulation.* 2000;101: 356–359.
28. Konertz W, Hotz H, Schneider M et al. Clinical experience with the MEDOS HIA-VAD system in infants and children. *Ann Thorac Surg.*1997; 63:1138–1144.
29. Ishino K, Loebe M, Uhlemann F et al. Circulatory support with paracorporeal pneumatic ventricular assist device (VAD) in infants and chidren. *Euro J Cardiothorac Surg.* 1997;11: 965–972.
30. Hetzer R, Potapov, Stiller B et al. Improvement in survival after mechanical circulatory support with pneumatic pulsatile ventricular assist devices in pediatric patients. *Ann Thorac Surg.* 2006;82:917–925.
31. Reinhartz O, Hill JD, Al-Khaldi A et al. Thoratec ventricular assist devices in pediatric patients: update on clinical results. *ASAIO J.*2005; 51:501–503.
32. Reinhartz O, Copeland JG, Farrar DJ. Thoratec ventricular assist devices in children with less than 1.3 m2 of body surface area. *ASAIO J.*2003; 49:727–730.
33. Blume ED, Naftel DC, Bastardi HJ et al. Pediatric Heart Transplant Study Investigators. Outcomes of children bridged to heart transplantation with ventricular assist devices: a multi-institutional study. *Circulation.*2006; 113:2313–2319.
34. O'Connor MJ, Menteer J, Chrisant MR et al. Ventricular assist device-associated anti-human leukocyte antigen antibody sensitization in pediatric patients bridged to heart transplantation. *J Heart Lung Transplant.*2010; 29:109–116.
35. Helman DN, Addonizio LJ, Morales DLS et al. Implantable left ventricular assist devices can successfully bridge adolescent patients to transplant. *J Heart Lung Transplant.* 2000;19: 121–126.
36. Chai PJ, Williamson A, Lodge AJ et al. Effects of ischemia on pulmonary dysfunction after cardiopulmonary bypass. *Ann Thorac Surg.*1999; 69:731–735.
37. Jaggers JJ, Forbess J, Shah A et al. Extracorporeal membrane oxygenation (ECMO) for post-cardiotomy failure in children: significance of shunt management in the single ventricle. *Ann Thorac Surg.*2000; 69: 1476–1483.
38. Hintz SR, Benitz WE, Colby CE et al. Utilization and outcomes of neonatal cardiac extracorporeal life support: 1996–2000. *Pediatr Crit Care Med.*2005; 6:33–38.
39. Ravishankar C, Dominguez TE, Kreutzer J et al. Extracorporeal membrane oxygenation after the Norwood Operation for hypoplastic left heart syndrome. *Pediatr Crit Care Med.* 2006;7:319–323.
40. Allan CK, Thiagarajan RR, del Nido PJ et al. Indication for initiation of mechanical circulatory support impacts survival of infants with shunted single-ventricle circulation supported with extracorporeal membrane oxygenation. *J Thorac Cardiovasc Surg.*2007; 133:660–667.

41. Ungerleider RM, Shen I, Yeh T et al. Routine mechanical ventricular assist following the Norwood procedure-improved neurologic outcome and excellent hospital survival. *Ann Thorac Surg*.2004 ;77: 18–22.
42. Booth KL, Roth SJ, Thiagarajan RR et al. Extracorporeal membrane oxygenation support of the Fontan and bidirectional Glenn circulations. *Ann Thorac Surg*.2004; 77:1341–1348.
43. Myers CD, Mattix K, Presson RG Jr et al. Twenty-four hour cardiopulmonary stability in a model of assisted newborn Fontan circulation. *Ann Thorac Surg*.2006; 81:264–270.
44. Throckmorton AL, Kishore RA. Design of a protective cage for an intravascular axial flow blood pump to mechanically assist the failing Fontan. *Artif Organ*.2009; 33:611–621.
45. Lacour-Gayet FG, Lanning CJ, Stoica S et al. An artificial right ventricle for failing fontan: in vitro and computational study. *Ann Thorac Surg*.2009; 88:170–176.
46. Ibrahim AE, Duncan BW, Blume ED et al. Long-term follow-up of pediatric cardiac patients requiring mechanical circulatory support. *Ann Thorac Surg*.2000; 69:186–192.
47. Rockett SR, Bryant JC, Morrow WR et al. Preliminary single center North American experience with the Berlin Heart pediatric EXCOR device. *ASAIO J*.2008; 54:479–482.
48. Russo P, Wheeler A, Russo J, Tobias JD. Use of a ventricular assist device as a bridge to transplantation in a patient with single ventricle physiology and total cavopulmonary anastomosis. *Paediatr Anaesth*.2008; 18:320–324.

Electrophysiology Issues and Heart Failure inC ongenitalH eartD isease

8

Scott R. Ceresnak and Anne M. Dubin

8.1 Introduction

There are two major causes of morbidity and mortality in children with heart failure: arrhythmia and pump failure.[1–4] Even in patients receiving treatment for their heart failure, pre-transplant mortality has been shown to be between 12% and 25%, with 25% of deaths secondary to an arrhythmia. The pediatric electrophysiologist can now offer therapies that address both causes of mortality, and potentially improve both quality of life and functional capacity.

Abnormalities in the heart rhythm are a relatively common occurrence in children with heart failure. In the patient with congenital heart disease and heart failure, both atrial and ventricular arrhythmias are frequently seen. These arrhythmias may either result from or lead to further destabilization of the underlying hemodynamic status. Assigning cause and effect can be extremely difficult in this situation.

In children, the spectrum of both pump failure and arrhythmias is different than in the adult population. Many therapies and treatment goals which have been extrapolated from the adult experience do not, in fact, translate well to the pediatric population. Prime examples of this are the treatment of atrial flutter and atrial fibrillation, and the role of implantable cardioverter-defibrillators (ICDs) and cardiac resynchronization therapy (CRT) in the adult, where the treatment in the adult ischemic population is markedly different than in pediatric patients with congenital heart disease.

In this chapter we will review the diagnosis and therapy of rhythm disturbances in pediatric patients with heart failure and discuss electrophysiologic treatment options for improvinghe modynamics.

S.R.C eresnak(✉)
Lucile Packard Children's Hospital, Stanford University School of Medicine,
Palo Alto, CA

R.E. Shaddy (ed.), *Heart Failure in Congenital Heart Disease*,
DOI: 10.1007/978-1-84996-480-7_8, © Springer-Verlag London Limited 2011

8.2
Arrhythmias in Children with Congenital Heart Disease and Heart Failure

Arrhythmias are a common finding in patients with congenital heart disease and heart failure.[5–10] Arrhythmias in heart failure may be the underlying cause of the heart failure, as in the case of tachycardia-induced cardiomyopathy, or may develop secondary to the ventricular dysfunction or anatomic abnormality.

8.2.1
Etiology of Arrhythmias

Patients with congenital heart disease and heart failure have multiple reasons for developing arrhythmias. Elevated end-diastolic pressures can lead to atrial or ventricular stretch.[11,12] Prior surgery with resultant atrial and ventricular scars can lead to an arrhythmogenic focus or provide the substrate for macro-reentrant tachycardia circuits.[13] Poor myocardial perfusion resulting from coronary lesions, and leading to ischemia serves as a substrate for arrhythmogenesis. Atrial or ventricular tissue may be structurally abnormal compared to the tissue in normal hearts and may provide the substrate for areas of abnormal conduction.[14] There are also multiple triggers for arrhythmia in patients with congenital heart disease and heart failure, which include abnormal electrolytes, blood gases and pH, as well as administration of potential pro-arrhythmic drugs.[15,16]

8.2.2
Atrial Arrhythmias

The ramifications of an atrial arrhythmia in the child with heart failure can be severe. In normal individuals, approximately 10–20% of cardiac output can be attributed to atrial augmentation of ventricular filling.[17] In patients with pre-existing ventricular dysfunction, loss of atrioventricular synchrony as a result of an atrial arrhythmia can lead to acute hemodynamic decompensation. The loss of atrioventricular synchrony can be exacerbated by significant elevation in resting heart rate which in turn leads to diminished diastolic filling time and therefore to diminished cardiac output. A prompt, correct diagnosis is therefore essential to restoration of sinus rhythm to improve the hemodynamic state of the patient.

8.2.2.1
Atrio-Ventricular Reentry Tachycardia (AVRT) and Atrio-Ventricular Nodal Reentry Tachycardia (AVNRT)

AVRT and AVNRT are the most common forms of supra-ventricular arrhythmias seen in the pediatric population.[18] While AVNRT is the more common of the two arrhythmias in adults, AVRT is the more common in infants, children, and adolescents, accounting for 73% of cases of supraventricular tachycardia (SVT).[18,19] Specific congenital anomalies have a predisposition to developing these arrhythmias. Patients with Ebstein's anomaly of the tricuspid valve and patients with hypertrophic cardiomyopathy are commonly affected. Thirty percent of patients with Ebstein's anomaly and 5% of patients with hypertrophic cardiomyopathy will have WPW and/or concealed retrograde conduction accessory pathways that place them at risk for the development of AVRT.[20,21]

8.2.2.2
Intra-Atrial Reentry Tachycardia (IART), Atrial Flutter, and Atrial Fibrillation (AFIB)

Intra-atrial reentry tachycardia (IART), atrial flutter, and atrial fibrillation (AFIB) are common in patients with heart failure. Etiologies include atrial stretch secondary to elevated filling pressures, and regions of conduction block due to surgical incision of the atrium in patients with a history of congenital heart disease and prior surgical repair.[12,22] Surgical incisions may lead to damage to normal atrial conduction tissue leading to areas of delayed atrial conduction and the propensity for re-entrant tachycardia.[23] These atrial tachyarrhythmias are especially common in patients with functional single ventricles after Fontan palliation, d-transposition of the great arteries after Mustard and Senning procedures, and patients with tetralogy of Fallot after surgical repair.[22–24] IART will occur in 50% of patients after Mustard or Senning procedures and up to 50% of patients who have undergone Fontan palliation.[25,26] Risk factors for development of late atrial arrhythmias in patients after the Fontan procedure include older age at repair, increased right atrial size, and elevated mean pulmonary artery pressures pre-operatively.[27]

8.2.2.3
Sinus Node Dysfunction

While patients with normal ventricular function can augment cardiac output by increasing stroke volume and increasing heart rate, these mechanisms are depleted in heart failure and many patients with heart failure and ventricular dysfunction rely on an increase in heart rate to increase cardiac output. The presence of sinus node dysfunction can thus further impair the ability of the patient with heart failure to augment cardiac output. In addition, patients with slow junctional rhythm with loss of atrial synchrony can have further worsening of heart failure symptoms. Sinus node dysfunction is common in patients who have undergone the Fontan operation and in patients who have undergone Mustard and Senning procedures. After the Fontan procedure, up to 45% of patients will exhibit abnormalities in sinus node function.[28,29] Loss of sinus rhythm after the Mustard procedure has been shown to occur in up to 23% of patients after 5 years and in up to 60% of patients after 20 years.[30] Possible etiologies of sinus node dysfunction include surgical damage to the sinus node, damage to the perinodal fibers surrounding the sinus node, and surgical disruption of blood flow to the sinus node artery.[23,30,31]

8.2.2.4
Ectopic Atrial Tachycardia and Multifocal Atrial Tachycardia

Patients with ectopic atrial tachycardia often present with cardiomyopathy as a result of their rhythm disturbance (Fig. 8.1).[32–34] Patients with primary cardiomyopathies, though, are also at heightened risk of developing ectopic atrial tachycardia. In the adult population, as many as 35% of patients with ventricular dysfunction and heart failure also have atrial tachycardia and atrial fibrillation.[35] It can be difficult to determine cause and effect in these situations.

Walsh et al. demonstrated that in young patients with ventricular dysfunction secondary to drug-resistant EAT, over 90% of patients can be cured with RF ablation and ventricular function can be expected to return to normal.[34] Thus, in a patient presenting with heart failure it is important to consider the possibility of tachycardia-induced cardiomyopathy, as this is a treatable and reversible cause of myocardial dysfunction.

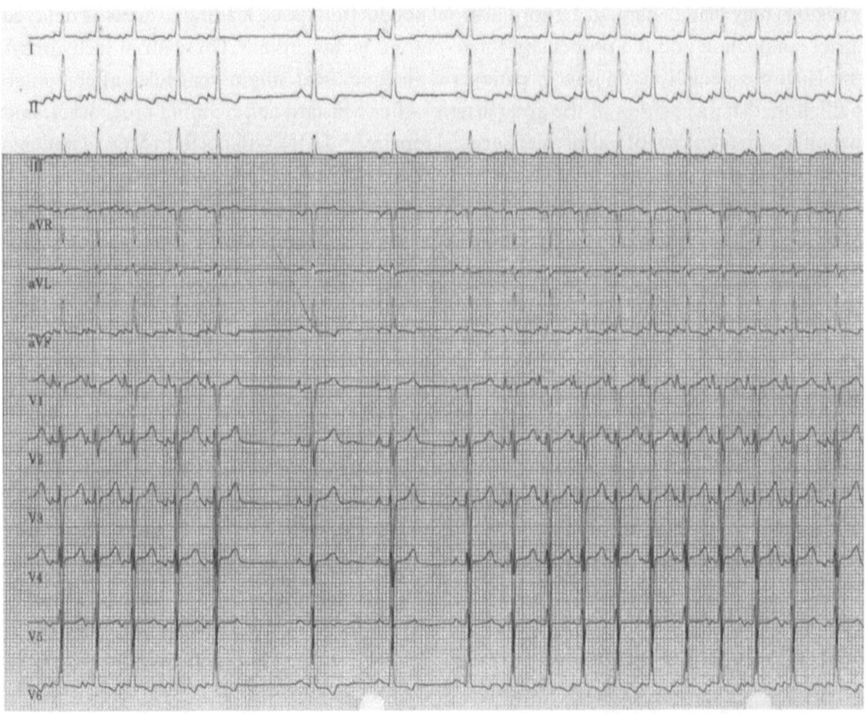

Fig. 8.1 Twelve lead electrocardiogram of 11 years old with incessant atrial tachycardia and poor function. ECG demonstrates break in tachycardia to slow sinus rhythm and re-initiation of atrial tachycardia with abnormal p wave and characteristic warm-up. Patient underwent ablation with recoveryofve ntricularf unction

8.2.3 Ventricular Arrhythmias

Ventricular arrhythmias are common in patients with heart failure and congenital heart disease. Ventricular tachycardia (VT) in these patients can develop as a consequence of prior surgical repair and incision within ventricular muscle, or may be secondary to residual hemodynamic impairment. Ventricular arrhythmias are common in patients with tetralogy of Fallot as well as left ventricular outflow tract obstructive lesions.[36,37] In patients with tetralogy of Fallot, the incidence of late VT has been reported to be 11.9% and the risk of sudden death has been reported at 8.3% by 35 years.[7]

The etiologies of VT in the heart failure population are as diverse as the underlying diagnoses. Poor myocardial perfusion in the setting of severe ventricular dysfunction may lead to ischemia and ventricular dysrhythmias. Scarring due to chronic ischemia, surgical incisions, or underlying abnormalities in the myocardium (such as patients with arrhythmogenic right ventricular cardiomyopathy and hypertrophic cardiomyopathy) may also serve as a nidus for arrhythmia.[13] Infection and myocarditis, leading to myocardial inflammation can lead to myocardial excitability.[38] Finally, intravenous catecholamines such as epinephrine, dopamine, or dobutamine administered for hemodynamic support can cause both atrial and ventricular arrhythmias. Although milrinone has been demonstrated to be arrhythmogenic in the adult population, there may be a lower incidence of arrhythmias seen in the pediatric population.[39]

8.2.4 Arrhythmia Therapies

8.2.4.1 Acute Therapy

Acute treatment is needed in the patient with a rapid atrial arrhythmia as well as those with a sustained VT. Patients who are unstable require immediate cardioversion or defibrillation.[40] Patients with congenital heart disease and heart failure require prompt restoration of sinus rhythm, as the tachyarrhythmia may not be tolerated for sustained periods of time. Adenosine can be used to terminate re-entrant rhythms such AVRT or AVNRT.

Atrial arrhythmias with rapid ventricular response rate may need acute therapy with atrioventricular nodal blocking agents. Digoxin, esmolol and diltiazem have all been used in this setting. Both diltiazem and esmolol must be used with caution as hypotension and decreased ventricular function can be seen with these drugs, especially in the setting of heart failure. The atrial rhythm itself may respond to IV procainamide or amiodarone. Again caution must be taken as both of these drugs can lead to hypotension. First line therapy for VT include lidocaine and amiodarone.

8.2.4.2
Chronic Therapy

Medications

Choice of anti-arrhythmic agents is limited in the setting of poor ventricular function. Beta blockers, with negative inotropic and chronotropic effects, often are not well tolerated in patients with acute decompensated heart failure. Class 1 agents such as procainamide and flecainide may lead to worsening ventricular function. Some care givers avoid flecainide in patients with congenital heart disease, poor ventricular function and VT. The CAST (Cardiac Arrhythmia Suppression Trial) study demonstrated increased morality in adults with ventricular arrhythmias following myocardial infarction.[41] This landmark study led to an avoidance of Class IC agents in patients with poor function and arrhythmias. Fish and colleagues investigated the use of IC agents in pediatric patients.[42] They found an increased risk of sudden death in pediatric patients with poor function and underlying heart disease. Amiodarone can be used safely in those with ventricular dysfunction as it may cause less hemodynamic embarrassment.[43] In addition, amiodarone has a high success rate for arrhythmia conversion and little pro-arrhythmic effects in children.[44]

8.2.4.3
Ablation Therapy

Catheter ablation is a commonly used modality of treatment for arrhythmias in children. Ablation therapy for atrial arrhythmias is safe and effective for children with structurally normal hearts.[45] Ablation can also be used with similar efficacy for specific arrhythmias in patients with congenital heart disease.[46] Catheter treatment of VT, however, is plagued by lower success rates and is less effective than for atrial arrhythmias.[47]

Patients with either ectopic atrial tachycardia (EAT) or tachycardia-induced cardiomyopathy may particularly benefit from catheter ablation. Walsh et al. demonstrated that in patients with ventricular dysfunction secondary to drug-resistant EAT, over 90% of patients can be cured with radiofrequency ablation and ventricular function should return to normal.[34]

Treatment of IART or atrial flutter may be more challenging. Ablation therapy in the adult population with atrial flutter most often involves ablation of the cavo-tricuspid isthmus and is acutely successful in 83% of patients.[48] Ablation success rates for IART in children with congenital heart disease has a much lower acute success rate (50% in patients with Fontan procedures) with a recurrence rate of 50%, often with different re-entry circuits.[49] In patients who have undergone Senning or Mustard procedures, more typical atrial flutter circuits are seen, which tend to be more amenable to ablation, with reported success rates of 70%.[50,51] The improved overall success rates and lower recurrence rates seen in patients following an atrial switch procedure as opposed to those who have had a Fontan procedure are thought to be secondary to less atrial hypertrophy.

Studies in adults with tetralogy of Fallot and VT have shown benefit from transcatheter VT ablation.[13] The VT in tetralogy of Fallot often involves a clockwise or counterclockwise circuit around the right ventricular outflow tract patch.[13,52] The placement of ablation lines from the right ventricular outflow tract patch to the tricuspid annulus and to the pulmonary annulus can lead to a cure of VT in 91% of patients.[13] The role of catheter ablation in younger patients remains less clearly defined.

8.2.4.4
Surgical Therapy

Surgical intervention may be warranted in the patient with frequent or intractable arrhythmias. Surgery may serve one of two roles: to improve the underlying patient hemodynamics leading to a decrease in the tachycardia substrate, or a therapeutic function of surgical arrhythmia ablation.

Two subsets of patients may particularly benefit from surgical intervention: patients with a univentricular heart who have undergone the Fontan procedure and patients with tetralogy of Fallot. As many as 50% of patients who have undergone a Fontan procedure will experience episodes of atrial tachycardia.[25] These arrhythmias, specifically IART, can lead to poor function and a significant decrease in quality of life. Radiofrequency ablation while relatively non-invasive has shown limited success with acute success of 50% and recurrences in approximately 50% of patients within 6 months.[53,54] Surgical conversion of Fontan patients with an atrio-pulmonary connection to a lateral tunnel or external conduit connection with concomitant Maze procedure has resulted in improved functional status as well as a decrease in atrial arrhythmias.[55]

Those patients with tetralogy of Fallot who have chronic volume load on the right ventricle with resultant right ventricular dilation, poor right ventricular function, and elevation of right ventricular pressures may be especially prone to VT and sudden death. Surgical intervention with placement of a pulmonary valve may decrease the risk of arrhythmias.[7,56] In adults, surgical placement of a pulmonary valve and surgical or transcatheter ablation has been shown in at least one series to decrease the recurrence of VT.[13,57]

8.2.4.5
Device Therapy

The use of ICDs has been demonstrated to prevent sudden cardiac death in adults with heart failure: the AVID trial demonstrated that adults who have survived a life threatening event have a reduction in mortality with an ICD compared to anti-arrhythmic pharmacotherapy.[58] Multiple trials in adults with poor ventricular function of varying etiologies have shown that ICD therapy is a powerful tool to decrease mortality. In the SCD-HeFT (Sudden Cardiac Death in Heart Failure) Trial, patients with an ejection fraction less than 35% and NYHA heart failure class III or IV[59] were randomized to receive conventional medical therapy plus amiodarone, ICD, or placebo. Patients in the ICD group were noted to have a reduction of mortality of 23% compared to the other groups. The group receiving amiodarone had no change in mortality when compared to the placebo group. Thus, ICD therapy is considered standard therapy for reducing the risk of sudden death in selected adult patients with heart failure.

There have been many small studies in pediatrics assessing the role of ICDs in children.[60–64] A recent, large, multi-center, retrospective study has shown that ICDs can be used safely and effectively in children.[63] In this study, 443 patients had ICDs placed and nearly 70% had a history of congenital heart disease with the most common diagnosis being tetralogy of Fallot (19%). Half of the ICDs placed were for primary prevention while the other half were implanted following an aborted sudden death episode or a syncopal episode. Twenty-six percent of patients had an appropriate shock. Inappropriate shocks were common as well, occurring in 21% of the patients. Inappropriate shocks occurred more commonly in the CHD population (28%) versus the cardiomyopathy population (13%).

ICDs have also been shown to serve as an effective bridge to transplant in both the adult and pediatric populations.[61,65,66] In adults, 1-year mortality while awaiting transplant is as high as 24%, and up to 30% of deaths occur suddenly secondary to an arrhythmia.[65,66] In adults, use of an ICD can significantly decrease mortality prior to transplantation.[65,66] In a study of 28 pediatric patients with ICDs placed while awaiting transplant, 46% of patients received an appropriate shock and complications in this group were low.[61]

Indications for ICD Placement

Indications for ICD placement in the pediatric population are based on adult data and limited pediatric data. The use of ICD's for secondary prevention has been generally well-established in the pediatric population; however, this can be difficult when dealing with the small patient (see below). The decision whether to place an ICD for primary prevention presents a more difficult challenge. Congenital heart lesions that are particularly susceptible to VT and sudden cardiac death are tetralogy of Fallot, d-transposition of the great arteries following a Mustard or Senning repair, congenital aortic stenosis and associated left ventricular outflow tract obstruction variants.[67]

Tetralogyo f Fallot

Sudden cardiac death occurs in patients late after repair of tetralogy of Fallot. The annual mortality for patients with tetralogy of Fallot is estimated to be 0.3%.[67] Several studies have been performed in the pediatric and young adult populations and have identified operative, hemodynamic and echocardiographic predictors of risk.[7,36,56,68–71] Surgical factors such as older age at initial repair, a history of a prior aortopulmonary shunt, the use of a trans-annular patch, a history of a ventriculotomy, and a history of early transient heart block have all been implicated in increasing the risk of sudden death. Hemodynamic factors including elevated right ventricular pressures, and a volume overloaded right ventricle, have also been shown to increase risk. Risk stratification has been attempted using QRS duration of >180 ms as a marker of a dilated poorly functioning right ventricle. Electrophysiologic ventricular stimulation studies can be useful, but the positive predictive value remains low at 55% and a negative study provides only limited reassurance.[72] There is general agreement that clinical symptoms and VT warrant aggressive investigation of hemodynamics and the consideration of ICD or ablation therapy.

d-Transposition of the Great Arteries After Mustard or Senning Procedures

As in patients with tetralogy of Fallot, patients with d-transposition of the great arteries who have a history of an atrial level switch procedure, either the Mustard or Senning procedure, are at increased risk of sudden death.[67,73] The incidence of sudden death in both children and adults has been shown to be as high as 10%.[30,74,75] The incidence of arrhythmias, including sinus node dysfunction, atrial flutter, and VT are all frequent occurrences and likely contribute to a sudden arrhythmogenic death. Though there is limited data on sudden death in this population, Kammarand and colleagues identified 47 young adult patients who experienced a sudden death event and had a history of atrial tachyarrhythmias.[76] These investigators found that heart failure and a history of symptoms associated with arrhythmias were predictors of sudden death. Interestingly, 81% of events occurred during exercise. This data suggests that atrial arrhythmias with rapid conduction lead to ventricular arrhythmias and collapse.

ICD Placement, Safety, and Testing

A recent, large, multi-center, retrospective study has shown that ICDs can be used safely and effectively in children.[63] Risks for devices in children appear to be slightly greater than in the adult population.[77] The risk of infection may be higher in children and in patients with congenital heart disease. Link and colleagues found that the risk of infection was significantly higher in pediatric patients than in adult patients (18% vs 1%).It also appears that patients with congenital heart disease have a higher incidence of lead infection when compared to those with structurally normal hearts. Klug and colleagues reviewed all patients less than 40 with pacemakers. They found a significant difference in pacemaker lead infections when comparing patients with (5.5%) and those without (2.3%) congenital heart disease.[78] While this study does not address ICD leads per se, it does support the premise that congenital heart disease itself is a complicating factor in device therapy.

Lead failure is higher in the pediatric population as well. Greater activity levels and a higher percent of epicardial leads have lead to 5-year lead failure and fracture rates as high as 15%.[63,79] This lead failure can be especially devastating in patients with ICDs as it often manifests as inappropriate ICD discharges. Pediatric patients with congenital heart disease are at higher risk for an inappropriate ICD discharge due to sinus tachycardia, oversensing, and lead fracture.[63,64] Approximately 16% of adults will experience an inappropriate discharge, while 21–25% of children will do so (Fig. 8.2).[63,64,80] Alexander and colleagues reviewed ICD therapy in 90 patients with either pediatric heart disease or congenital heart disease.[64] They found the majority of inappropriate ICD discharges in children occurred secondary to lead failure. Interestingly, patient size and age did not predict lead failure, but rapid growth did.

Venous occlusion is also a potential complication of transvenous systems. Venous occlusion is found in 15–21% of all pediatric patients with ICD or pacemaker leads.[81,82] Transvenous placement of ICD may be limited secondary to small size, risk of venous occlusion and venous or cardiac anatomy. Presently there have been multiple institutions which have utilized epicardial and novel configurations of ICD leads.[83–85] These new and

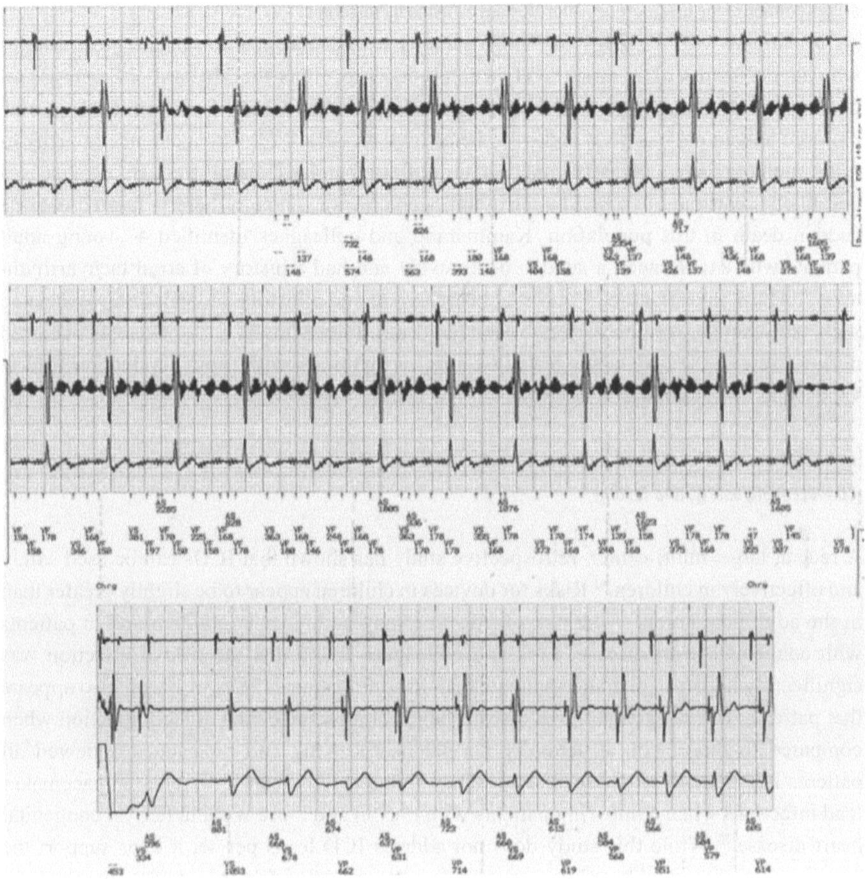

Fig. 8.2 Fifteen years old with implantable cardioverter defibrillator following near sudden death episode with an inappropriate discharge. Patient was exposed to electrical interference, which was interpreted by the device as ventricular tachycardia/fibrillation with resulting defibrillation

novel methods have been found to be quite effective with good defibrillation thresholds in individualpa tients.

8.3 Hemodynamic Management Strategies

8.3.1 Cardiac Resynchronization Therapy (CRT)

CRT is a relatively new pacing modality that can be employed as a therapeutic option for patients with heart failure, ventricular dyssynchrony, and diminished left ventricular function. In patients with mechanical and/or electrical dyssynchrony, pacing both the right and left ventricles can improve hemodynamics and diminish patient symptoms by augmenting cardiac output.

In structurally normal hearts with intact conduction systems, the spread of electrical energy through the atrioventricular node, His-Purkinje system, and the right and left bundle branches leads to synchronous right and left ventricular contraction. The presence of conduction system abnormalities, such as a bundle branch block and a widened QRS on surface ECG, can lead to impairment in the usual synchronous ventricular contraction.[86,87] This electrical dyssynchrony becomes especially important in those with impaired ventricular function.

A number of large, randomized studies of CRT have shown marked improvement in symptoms and function in adults with dyssynchrony and heart failure. The MIRACLE (Multicenter Insync Randomized Clinical Evaluation), MUSTIC (Multi-site Stimulation in Cardiomyopathies), and COMPANION (Comparison of Medical Therapy Pacing and Defibrillation in Heart Failure) trials have demonstrated improved quality of life, exercise tolerance and functional status.[88–90] Most importantly, the COMPANION trial demonstrated a 20% reduction in mortality with CRT compared with optimization of medical therapy and a 36% reduction in mortality with CRT/ICD therapy versus optimal medical therapy.[89]

In the adult population, CRT is indicated for patients with NYHA class III or IV heart failure, a wide QRS greater than 120 ms, and a left ventricular ejection fraction less than 35% despite optimal medical therapy.[91] However, in the pediatric population, few patients will meet the adult criteria.[92] Pediatric patients have been shown to benefit from CRT, but determining which patients will benefit requires a different set of guidelines than the adult population. Multiple small pediatric studies have shown that CRT can be beneficial in a variety of pediatric patients who do not fit the adult criteria, including patients with congenital heart disease. CRT has been studied in both left and right ventricular failure and in patients with single ventricle physiology. In eight pediatric patients with systemic right ventricular failure, Janousek demonstrated a decrease in interventricular mechanical delay and improvement in right ventricular ejection fraction with CRT.[93] Dubin et al. evaluated seven patients with congenital heart disease, subpulmonary right ventricular dysfunction, and a right bundle branch block, and demonstrated an improved cardiac index and right ventricular dP/dt along with a decreased QRS duration.[94] Strieper and colleagues investigated post-operative use of CRT in seven patients following repair of congenital heart disease with biventricular repairs and noted improvement in LV dimensions and improved ejection fraction. Five of the seven patients in that series improved significantly enough to be removed from the cardiac transplant list.[95] In patients with univentricular hearts, Zimmerman and colleagues noted that in 26 patients, CRT led to improvement in systolic blood pressure, echocardiographic mechanical synchrony, and cardiac index.[96,97] Recently Cecchin and colleagues reported on 60 patients who underwent CRT from a single institution, of which 13 had single ventricle physiology. They found improvement in NYHA classification in eleven of the thirteen as well as improved ejection fraction in 10.[98] The largest series of CRT in children was a retrospective, multi-center report by Dubin and colleagues. In that series, 103 patients were evaluated and 71% were noted to have congenital heart disease. CRT was noted to be associated with a significant reduction in QRS

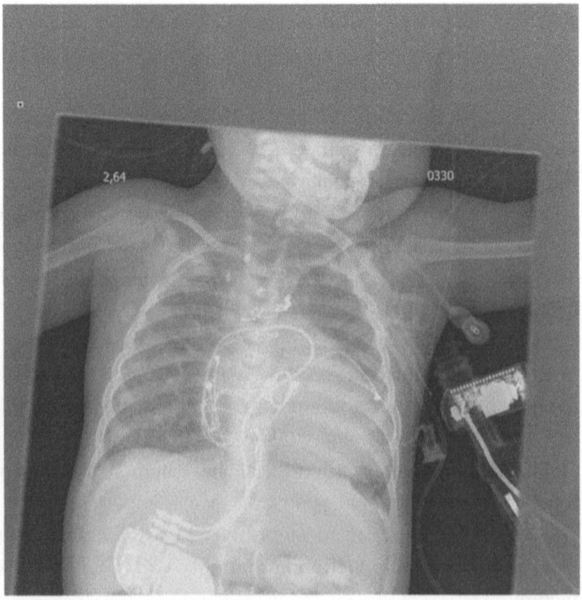

Fig. 8. 3 Twentymonthol d child with mitral valve replacement, poor ventricular function and congenital complete heart block, after implantation of epicardial biventricular pacemaker

duration, increased systemic ventricular ejection fraction, and, in three patients, improvement in hemodynamics enough to avoid cardiac transplantation. Thus, though indications are different in the pediatric population, pediatric patients can also benefit from CRT.

Lead placement may also be more challenging in the pediatric and congenital heart disease population compared to the adult population. Pediatric patients have smaller vessels which are more prone to thrombosis and occlusion.[81,82] Fifty-eight percent of the resynchronization devices placed in the international pediatric study were epicardial or mixed systems as opposed to the usual 5% of adult systems (Fig. 8.3).[88,99] In the MIRACLE trial, 12% of adult patients had issues related to coronary sinus lead placement compared to 18% in pediatric patients who had a lead placed in a transvenous fashion.[88,99] This discrepancy may be related to patient size, increased presence of congenital heart disease in the pediatric population, and operator experience.

8.4 Conclusion and Future Considerations

Arrhythmias are a major contributor to morbidity and mortality in pediatric patients with congenital heart disease and heart failure. Anti-arrhythmic agents, electrophysiologic interventions, and device therapy can all help reduce the risk of arrhythmia in this population. Unfortunately it can be quite difficult to assess risk prior to any development of arrhythmia. Further work in risk stratification is needed in this population.

Recently a new device therapy, CRT has been shown to be beneficial in improving hemodynamics at least in some patients with congenital heart disease. Further work in who would benefit and how to best institute this therapy is necessary in the pediatric population.

References

1. Steinberger J, Haines HC, Shumway SJ, Bolman RM, 3rd, Rocchini AP, Braunlin EA. Outcome after referral for pediatric transplantation. *J Heart Lung Transplant.* 1993;12: 766–769.
2. Rosenthal DN, Dubin AM, Chin C, Falco D, Gamberg P, Bernstein D. Outcome while awaiting heart transplantation in children: a comparison of congenital heart disease and cardiomyopathy. *J Heart Lung Transplant.*2000; 19:751–755.
3. Nield LE, McCrindle BW, Bohn DJ et al. Outcomes for children with cardiomyopathy awaiting transplantation. *Cardiol Young.*2000; 10:358–366.
4. Morrow WR, Frazier E, Naftel DC. Survival after listing for cardiac transplantation in children. *Prog Pediatr Cardiol.*2000; 11:99–105.
5. Gillette PC, Yeoman MA, Mullins CE, McNamara DG. Sudden death after repair of tetralogy of Fallot. Electrocardiographic and electrophysiologic abnormalities. *Circulation.* 1977;56: 566–571.
6. Friedman RA, Moak JP, Garson A, Jr. Clinical course of idiopathic dilated cardiomyopathy in children. *J Am Coll Cardiol.*1991; 18:152–156.
7. Gatzoulis MA, Balaji S, Webber SA et al. Risk factors for arrhythmia and sudden cardiac death late after repair of tetralogy of Fallot: a multicentre study. *Lancet.*2000; 356:975–981.
8. Griffin ML, Hernandez A, Martin TC et al. Dilated cardiomyopathy in infants and children. *J Am Coll Cardiol.*1988; 11:139–144.
9. Hayes CJ, Gersony WM. Arrhythmias after the Mustard operation for transposition of the great arteries: a long-term study. *J Am Coll Cardiol.*1986; 7:133–137.
10. Lewis AB, Chabot M. Outcome of infants and children with dilated cardiomyopathy. *Am J Cardiol.*1991;68:3 65–369.
11. Franz MR, Bode F. Mechano-electrical feedback underlying arrhythmias: the atrial fibrillation case. *Prog Biophys Mol Biol.*2003; 82:163–174.
12. Vaziri SM, Larson MG, Benjamin EJ, Levy D. Echocardiographic predictors of nonrheumatic atrial fibrillation. The Framingham Heart Study. *Circulation.*1994; 89:724–730.
13. Zeppenfeld K, Schalij MJ, Bartelings MM et al. Catheter ablation of ventricular tachycardia after repair of congenital heart disease: electroanatomic identification of the critical right ventricular isthmus. *Circulation.*2007; 116:2241–2252.
14. Sanchez-Quintana D, Climent V, Ho SY, Anderson RH. Myoarchitecture and connective tissue in hearts with tricuspid atresia. *Heart.*1999; 81:182–191.
15. Dyckner T, Wester PO. Potassium/magnesium depletion in patients with cardiovascular disease. *Am J Med.*19 87;82:11–17.
16. Wiles HB, Gillette PC, Harley RA, Upshur JK. Cardiomyopathy and myocarditis in children with ventricular ectopic rhythm. *J Am Coll Cardiol.*1992; 20:359–362.
17. Samet P, Bernstein WH, Nathan DA, Lopez A. Atrial Contribution to Cardiac Output in Complete Heart Block. *Am J Cardiol.*1965; 16:1–10.
18. Ko JK, Deal BJ, Strasburger JF, Benson DW, Jr. Supraventricular tachycardia mechanisms and their age distribution in pediatric patients. *Am J Cardiol.*1992; 69:1028–1032.

19. Akhtar M, Jazayeri MR, Sra J, Blanck Z, Deshpande S, Dhala A. Atrioventricular nodal reentry. Clinical, electrophysiological, and therapeutic considerations. *Circulation*. 1993;88: 282–295.
20. Fananapazir L, Tracy CM, Leon MB et al. Electrophysiologic abnormalities in patients with hypertrophic cardiomyopathy. A consecutive analysis in 155 patients. *Circulation*. 1989;80: 1259–1268.
21. Vacca JB, Bussmann DW, Mudd JG. Ebstein's anomaly; complete review of 108 cases. *Am J Cardiol*.1958;2:210–226.
22. Abrams D, Schilling R. Mechanism and mapping of atrial arrhythmia in the modified Fontan circulation. *Heart Rhythm*.2005; 2:1138–1144.
23. Gillette PC, Kugler JD, Garson A, Jr., Gutgesell HP, Duff DF, McNamara DG. Mechanisms of cardiac arrhythmias after the Mustard operation for transposition of the great arteries. *Am J Cardiol*.1980;45 :1225–1230.
24. Roos-Hesselink J, Perlroth MG, McGhie J, Spitaels S. Atrial arrhythmias in adults after repair of tetralogy of Fallot. Correlations with clinical, exercise, and echocardiographic findings. *Circulation*.1995; 91:2214–2219.
25. Deal BJ, Mavroudis C, Backer CL. Arrhythmia management in the Fontan patient. *Pediatr Cardiol*.2007;28 :448–456.
26. Vetter VL, Tanner CS, Horowitz LN. Electrophysiologic consequences of the Mustard repair of d-transposition of the great arteries. *J Am Coll Cardiol*.1987; 10:1265–1273.
27. Gewillig M, Wyse RK, de Leval MR, Deanfield JE. Early and late arrhythmias after the Fontan operation: predisposing factors and clinical consequences. *Br Heart J*.1992; 67:72–79.
28. Manning PB, Mayer JE, Jr., Wernovsky G, Fishberger SB, Walsh EP. Staged operation to Fontan increases the incidence of sinoatrial node dysfunction. *J Thorac Cardiovasc Surg*. 1996;111:833–839; discussion 839–840.
29. Shah MJ, Nehgme R, Carboni M, Murphy JD. Endocardial atrial pacing lead implantation and midterm follow-up in young patients with sinus node dysfunction after the fontan procedure. *Pacing Clin Electrophysiol*.2004; 27:949–954.
30. Gelatt M, Hamilton RM, McCrindle BW et al. Arrhythmia and mortality after the Mustard procedure: a 30-year single-center experience. *J Am Coll Cardiol*.1997; 29:194–201.
31. Vetter VL, Tanner CS. Electrophysiologic consequences of the arterial switch repair of d-transposition of the great arteries. *J Am Coll Cardiol*.1988; 12:229–237.
32. Packer DL, Bardy GH, Worley SJ et al. Tachycardia-induced cardiomyopathy: a reversible form of left ventricular dysfunction. *Am J Cardiol*.198 6;57:563–570.
33. Horenstein MS, Saarel E, Dick M, Karpawich PP. Reversible symptomatic dilated cardiomyopathy in older children and young adolescents due to primary non-sinus supraventricular tachyarrhythmias. *Pediatr Cardiol*.2003; 24:274–279.
34. Walsh EP, Saul JP, Hulse JE et al. Transcatheter ablation of ectopic atrial tachycardia in young patients using radiofrequency current. *Circulation*.199 2;86:1138–1146.
35. Ozcan C, Jahangir A, Friedman PA et al. Long-term survival after ablation of the atrioventricular node and implantation of a permanent pacemaker in patients with atrial fibrillation. *N Engl J Med*.2001; 344:1043–1051.
36. Khairy P, Harris L, Landzberg MJ et al. Implantable cardioverter-defibrillators in tetralogy of Fallot. *Circulation*.2008; 117:363–370.
37. Minakata K, Dearani JA, O'Leary PW, Danielson GK. Septal myectomy for obstructive hypertrophic cardiomyopathy in pediatric patients: early and late results. *Ann Thorac Surg*. 2005;80:1424–1429; discussion 1429–1430.
38. Sharma JR, Sathanandam S, Rao SP, Acharya S, Flood V. Ventricular tachycardia in acute fulminant myocarditis: medical management and follow-up. *Pediatr Cardiol*. 2008;29: 416–419.

39. Hoffman TM, Wernovsky G, Atz AM et al. Efficacy and safety of milrinone in preventing low cardiac output syndrome in infants and children after corrective surgery for congenital heart disease. *Circulation.*2003; 107:996–1002.
40. Bossaert L, Van Hoeyweghen R. Bystander cardiopulmonary resuscitation (CPR) in out-of-hospital cardiac arrest. The Cerebral Resuscitation Study Group. *Resuscitation.* 1989;17(suppl): S55–S69; discussion S199–S206.
41. Preliminary report: effect of encainide and flecainide on mortality in a randomized trial of arrhythmia suppression after myocardial infarction. The Cardiac Arrhythmia Suppression Trial (CAST) Investigators. *N Engl J Med.*1989; 321:406–412.
42. Fish FA, Gillette PC, Benson DW, Jr. Proarrhythmia, cardiac arrest and death in young patients receiving encainide and flecainide. The Pediatric Electrophysiology Group. *J Am Coll Cardiol.* 1991;18:356–365.
43. Perry JC, Knilans TK, Marlow D, Denfield SW, Fenrich AL, Friedman RA. Intravenous amiodarone for life-threatening tachyarrhythmias in children and young adults. *J Am Coll Cardiol.* 1993;22:95–98.
44. Coumel P, Fidelle J. Amiodarone in the treatment of cardiac arrhythmias in children: one hundred thirty-five cases. *Am Heart J.*1980; 100:1063–1069.
45. Friedman RA, Walsh EP, Silka MJ et al. NASPE Expert Consensus Conference: Radiofrequency catheter ablation in children with and without congenital heart disease. Report of the writing committee. North American Society of Pacing and Electrophysiology. *Pacing Clin Electrophysiol.*200 2;25:1000–1017.
46. Van Hare GF, Lesh MD, Stanger P. Radiofrequency catheter ablation of supraventricular arrhythmias in patients with congenital heart disease: results and technical considerations. *J Am Coll Cardiol.*1993; 22:883–890.
47. Morwood JG, Triedman JK, Berul CI et al. Radiofrequency catheter ablation of ventricular tachycardia in children and young adults with congenital heart disease. *Heart Rhythm.* 2004;1:301–308.
48. Thornton AS, Janse P, Alings M et al. Acute success and short-term follow-up of catheter ablation of isthmus-dependent atrial flutter; a comparison of 8 mm tip radiofrequency and cryothermy catheters. *J Interv Card Electrophysiol.*2008; 21:241–248.
49. Triedman JK, Bergau DM, Saul JP, Epstein MR, Walsh EP. Efficacy of radiofrequency ablation for control of intraatrial reentrant tachycardia in patients with congenital heart disease. *J Am Coll Cardiol.*1997; 30:1032–1038.
50. Kanter RJ, Papagiannis J, Carboni MP, Ungerleider RM, Sanders WE, Wharton JM. Radiofrequency catheter ablation of supraventricular tachycardia substrates after mustard and senning operations for d-transposition of the great arteries. *J Am Coll Cardiol.* 2000;35: 428–441.
51. Van Hare GF, Lesh MD, Ross BA, Perry JC, Dorostkar PC. Mapping and radiofrequency ablation of intraatrial reentrant tachycardia after the Senning or Mustard procedure for transposition ofthe great arteries. *Am J Cardiol.*1996; 77:985–991.
52. Misaki T, Tsubota M, Watanabe G et al. Surgical treatment of ventricular tachycardia after surgical repair of tetralogy of Fallot. Relation between intraoperative mapping and histological findings. *Circulation.*1994; 90:264–271.
53. Triedman JK, Jenkins KJ, Colan SD, Saul JP, Walsh EP. Intra-atrial reentrant tachycardia after palliation of congenital heart disease: characterization of multiple macroreentrant circuits using fluoroscopically based three-dimensional endocardial mapping. *J Cardiovasc Electrophysiol.*199 7;8:259–270.
54. Triedman JK, Saul JP, Weindling SN, Walsh EP. Radiofrequency ablation of intra-atrial reentrant tachycardia after surgical palliation of congenital heart disease. *Circulation.* 1995;91: 707–714.

55. Mavroudis C, Backer CL, Deal BJ, Johnsrude CL. Fontan conversion to cavopulmonary connection and arrhythmia circuit cryoblation. *J Thorac Cardiovasc Surg*.1998; 115:547–556.
56. Zahka KG, Horneffer PJ, Rowe SA et al. Long-term valvular function after total repair of tetralogy of Fallot. Relation to ventricular arrhythmias. *Circulation*.1988; 78:III14–III19.
57. Therrien J, Siu SC, Harris L et al. Impact of pulmonary valve replacement on arrhythmia propensity late after repair of tetralogy of Fallot. *Circulation*.2001; 103:2489–2494.
58. A comparison of antiarrhythmic-drug therapy with implantable defibrillators in patients resuscitated from near-fatal ventricular arrhythmias. The Antiarrhythmics versus Implantable Defibrillators (AVID) Investigators. *N Engl J Med*.199 7;337:1576–1583.
59. Bardy GH, Lee KL, Mark DB et al. Amiodarone or an implantable cardioverter-defibrillator for congestive heart failure. *N Engl J Med*.2005; 352:225–237.
60. Hamilton RM, Dorian P, Gow RM, Williams WG. Five-year experience with implantable defibrillators in children. *Am J Cardiol*.1996; 77:524–526.
61. Dubin AM, Berul CI, Bevilacqua LM et al. The use of implantable cardioverter-defibrillators in pediatric patients awaiting heart transplantation. *J Card Fail*.2003; 9:375–379.
62. Silka MJ, Kron J, Dunnigan A, Dick M, 2nd. Sudden cardiac death and the use of implantable cardioverter-defibrillators in pediatric patients. The Pediatric Electrophysiology Society. *Circulation*.1993; 87:800–807.
63. Berul CI, Van Hare GF, Kertesz NJ et al. Results of a multicenter retrospective implantable cardioverter-defibrillator registry of pediatric and congenital heart disease patients. *J Am Coll Cardiol*.2008;51 :1685–1691.
64. Alexander ME, Cecchin F, Walsh EP, Triedman JK, Bevilacqua LM, Berul CI. Implications of implantable cardioverter defibrillator therapy in congenital heart disease and pediatrics. *J Cardiovasc Electrophysiol*.2004; 15:72–76.
65. Sandner SE, Wieselthaler G, Zuckermann A et al. Survival benefit of the implantable cardioverter-defibrillator in patients on the waiting list for cardiac transplantation. *Circulation*. 2001;104:I171–I176.
66. Schmidinger H. The implantable cardioverter defibrillator as a "bridge to transplant": a viable clinical strategy? *Am J Cardiol*.1999; 83:151D–157D.
67. Silka MJ, Hardy BG, Menashe VD, Morris CD. A population-based prospective evaluation of risk of sudden cardiac death after operation for common congenital heart defects. *J Am Coll Cardiol*.1998;32 :245–251.
68. Gatzoulis MA, Till JA, Somerville J, Redington AN. Mechanoelectrical interaction in tetralogy of Fallot. QRS prolongation relates to right ventricular size and predicts malignant ventricular arrhythmias and sudden death. *Circulation*.199 5;92:231–237.
69. Chandar JS, Wolff GS, Garson A, Jr. et al. Ventricular arrhythmias in postoperative tetralogy of Fallot. *Am J Cardiol*.1990; 65:655–661.
70. Harrison DA, Harris L, Siu SC et al. Sustained ventricular tachycardia in adult patients late after repair of tetralogy of Fallot. *J Am Coll Cardiol*.1997; 30:1368–1373.
71. Hokanson JS, Moller JH. Significance of early transient complete heart block as a predictor of sudden death late after operative correction of tetralogy of Fallot. *Am J Cardiol*. 2001;87: 1271–1277.
72. Khairy P, Landzberg MJ, Gatzoulis MA et al. Value of programmed ventricular stimulation after tetralogy of fallot repair: a multicenter study. *Circulation*.2004; 109:1994–2000.
73. Sarkar D, Bull C, Yates R et al. Comparison of long-term outcomes of atrial repair of simple transposition with implications for a late arterial switch strategy. *Circulation*. 1999;100: II176–II181.
74. Puley G, Siu S, Connelly M et al. Arrhythmia and survival in patients >18 years of age after the mustard procedure for complete transposition of the great arteries. *Am J Cardiol*. 1999;83: 1080–1084.
75. Dos L, Teruel L, Ferreira IJ et al. Late outcome of Senning and Mustard procedures for correction of transposition of the great arteries. *Heart*. 2005;91:652–656.

76. Kammeraad JA, van Deurzen CH, Sreeram N et al. Predictors of sudden cardiac death after Mustard or Senning repair for transposition of the great arteries. *J Am Coll Cardiol.* 2004;44:1095–1102.
77. Link MS, Hill SL, Cliff DL et al. Comparison of frequency of complications of implantable cardioverter-defibrillators in children versus adults. *Am J Cardiol.* 1999;83:263–266, A5–A6.
78. Klug D, Vaksmann G, Jarwe M et al. Pacemaker lead infection in young patients. *Pacing Clin Electrophysiol.*200 3;26:1489–1493.
79. Fortescue EB, Berul CI, Cecchin F, Walsh EP, Triedman JK, Alexander ME. Patient, procedural, and hardware factors associated with pacemaker lead failures in pediatrics and congenital heart disease. *Heart Rhythm.*2004; 1:150–159.
80. Grimm W, Menz V, Hoffmann J et al. Complications of third-generation implantable cardioverter defibrillator therapy. *Pacing Clin Electrophysiol.*1999; 22:206–211.
81. Figa FH, McCrindle BW, Bigras JL, Hamilton RM, Gow RM. Risk factors for venous obstruction in children with transvenous pacing leads. *Pacing Clin Electrophysiol.* 1997;20: 1902–1909.
82. Bar-Cohen Y, Berul CI, Alexander ME et al. Age, size, and lead factors alone do not predict venous obstruction in children and young adults with transvenous lead systems. *J Cardiovasc Electrophysiol.*200 6;17:754–759.
83. Stephenson EA, Batra AS, Knilans TK et al. A multicenter experience with novel implantable cardioverter defibrillator configurations in the pediatric and congenital heart disease population. *J Cardiovasc Electrophysiol.*2006; 17:41–46.
84. Bauersfeld U, Tomaske M, Dodge-Khatami A, Rahn M, Kellenberger CJ, Pretre R. Initial experience with implantable cardioverter defibrillator systems using epicardial and pleural electrodes in pediatric patients. *Ann Thorac Surg.*2007; 84:303–305.
85. Kriebel T, Ruschewski W, Gonzalez y Gonzalez M et al. ICD Implantation in infants and small children: the extracardiac technique. *Pacing Clin Electrophysiol.*2006; 29:1319–1325.
86. Grines CL, Bashore TM, Boudoulas H, Olson S, Shafer P, Wooley CF. Functional abnormalities in isolated left bundle branch block. The effect of interventricular asynchrony. *Circulation.* 1989;79:845–853.
87. Duncan AM, Francis DP, Gibson DG, Henein MY. Limitation of exercise tolerance in chronic heart failure: distinct effects of left bundle-branch block and coronary artery disease. *J Am Coll Cardiol.*2004 ;43:1524–1531.
88. Abraham WT, Fisher WG, Smith AL et al. Cardiac resynchronization in chronic heart failure. *N Engl J Med.*200 2;346:1845–1853.
89. Bristow MR, Saxon LA, Boehmer J et al. Cardiac-resynchronization therapy with or without an implantable defibrillator in advanced chronic heart failure. *N Engl J Med.* 2004;350: 2140–2150.
90. Cazeau S, Leclercq C, Lavergne T et al. Effects of multisite biventricular pacing in patients with heart failure and intraventricular conduction delay. *N Engl J Med.*2001; 344:873–880.
91. Epstein AE, Dimarco JP, Ellenbogen KA et al. ACC/AHA/HRS 2008 Guidelines for device-based therapy of cardiac rhythm abnormalities. *Heart Rhythm.*2008; 5:e1–e62.
92. Alexander ME, Berul CI, Fortescue EB et al. Who is eligible for cardiac resyncrhonization-therapy in pediatric cardiology? *Heart Rhythm.*2004; 1:S122.
93. Janousek J, Tomek V, Chaloupecky VA et al. Cardiac resynchronization therapy: a novel adjunct to the treatment and prevention of systemic right ventricular failure. *J Am Coll Cardiol.* 2004;44:1927–1931.
94. Dubin AM, Feinstein JA, Reddy VM, Hanley FL, Van Hare GF, Rosenthal DN. Electrical resynchronization: a novel therapy for the failing right ventricle. *Circulation.* 2003;107:2287–2289.
95. Strieper M, Karpawich P, Frias P et al. Initial experience with cardiac resynchronization therapy for ventricular dysfunction in young patients with surgically operated congenital heart disease. *Am J Cardiol.*2004; 94:1352–1354.

96. Bacha EA, Zimmerman FJ, Mor-Avi V et al. Ventricular resynchronization by multisite pacing improves myocardial performance in the postoperative single-ventricle patient. *Ann Thorac Surg*.2004; 78:1678–1683.
97. Zimmerman FJ, Starr JP, Koenig PR, Smith P, Hijazi ZM, Bacha EA. Acute hemodynamic benefit of multisite ventricular pacing after congenital heart surgery. *Ann Thorac Surg*. 2003;75:1775–1780.
98. Cecchin F, Frangini PA, Brown DW et al. Cardiac Resynchronization Therapy (and Multisite Pacing) in Pediatrics and Congenital Heart Disease: Five Years Experience in a Single Institution. *J Cardiovasc Electrophysiol*.2008; 58–65.
99. Dubin AM, Janousek J, Rhee E et al. Resynchronization therapy in pediatric and congenital heart disease patients: an international multicenter study. *J Am Coll Cardiol*. 2005;46: 2277–2283.

Index

I

J

K

L

M

N

O

MIX
Papier aus verantwortungsvollen Quellen
Paper from responsible sources
FSC® C105338

If you have any concerns about our products,
you can contact us on
ProductSafety@springernature.com

In case Publisher is established outside the EU,
the EU authorized representative is:
Springer Nature Customer Service Center GmbH
Europaplatz 3, 69115 Heidelberg, Germany

Printed by Libri Plureos GmbH
in Hamburg, Germany